G.I. Obrams   M. Potter (Eds.)

Epidemiology and Biology of Multiple Myeloma

With 30 Figures

Springer-Verlag
Berlin Heidelberg New York
London Paris Tokyo
Hong Kong Barcelona
Budapest

G. Iris Obrams, M. D., Ph. D.
Chief, Extramural Programs Branch
Epidemiology & Biostatistics Program
Division of Cancer Etiology, National Cancer Institute
Bethesda, MD 20892, USA

Michael Potter, M. D.
Chief, Laboratory of Genetics
Division of Cancer Biology, Diagnosis,
and Centers, National Cancer Institute
Bethesda, MD 20892, USA

ISBN-13: 978-3-642-76657-2 **e-ISBN-13: 978-3-642-76655-8**
DOI: 10.1007/ 978-3-642-76655-8

Library of Congress Cataloging-in-Publication Data

Softcover reprint of the hardcover 1st edition 1991

23/3145-543210 – Printed on acid-free paper

Dedication

The participants and contributors to this workshop dedicate this book to the memory of Elliott F. Osserman (1925–1989). His enthusiasm for the pursuit of clinical and scientific understanding of multiple myeloma was and still is an inspiration to many of us.

Elliott became one of the foremost clinical authorities on myeloma in the United States and his work in this field was recognized internationally. He took great pride in getting his patients through this difficult disease and extending their lives with comfort; he treated many well-known people in the New York area and beyond. But in addition to this committment to outstanding clinical medicine, Elliott continued to study in depth each of his cases of multiple myeloma looking for new clues about its origin and nature. It was during such an inquiry that he found an unusual protein in the urine of one of his patients that he identified as lysozyme. Actually this patient had developed a myelomonocytic leukemia that was secreting lysozyme. Elliott became fascinated with the relationship of the leukemia to the plasma cell and speculated the two processes might be associated with a common lineage. He devoted many of his later studies to its structure and biosynthesis of human lysozyme.

The picture of Elliott (right) and Jan Waldenstrom was taken when they both attended a myeloma workshop given in honor of Jan Waldenstrom at the NIH in 1980. I am sure Elliott would be pleased to be remembered beside of his great friend and colleague.

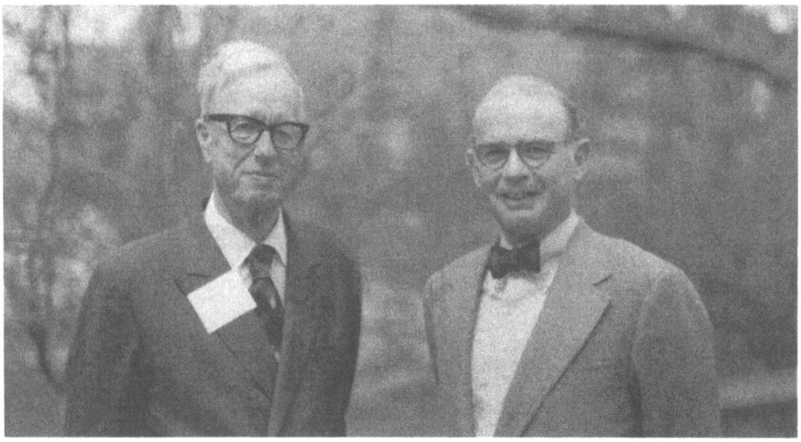

Preface

On March 27, 1990, the National Cancer Institute sponsored a workshop on the epidemiology of multiple myeloma, held at the National Institutes of Health. This book comprises articles prepared by participants in this workshop. Discussed in these papers are: the descriptive and analytic epidemiology, differences in risk factors between blacks and whites, monoclonal gammopathies and their progression, and hypotheses regarding the etiology and pathogenesis of multiple myeloma.

Several epidemiologic research areas received particular attention during this workshop, and are reviewed in detail in this volume. There have been striking increases in the incidence of multiple myeloma over the past thirty years, especially among older individuals and blacks, which may not be entirely explained by changes in diagnostic capabilities. Occupational and environmental exposures have been associated with an increased risk of multiple myeloma, including farming exposures, occupational exposure to petroleum and rubber processing, exposure to ionizing radiation, and associations with persistent virus infections. The most striking epidemiological finding is reflected in the differences in incidence rates of multiple myeloma which are twice as high in blacks as compared with whites. Further, since 1950 the mortality rates for multiple myeloma have quadrupled in blacks while doubling for whites. Among hematopoietic malignancies, multiple myeloma is the only one with increased incidence and mortality rates among blacks.

Two major possibilities for explaining ethnic/racial differences in susceptibility to multiple myeloma are genetic and environmental factors. The present studies have not implicated specific determinants for either of these two factors as yet. Limited studies available from African populations suggest that plasma cell dyscrasias may be as prevalent among African blacks as among American blacks, suggesting the importance of racial factors, but these peoples are also exposed to different sets of environmental factors. The relative importance of genetic and environmental factors will require careful attention in projected studies.

A major question concerns the relationship of monoclonal gammopathy of undetermined significance (MGUS) to multiple myeloma. MGUS can convert to myeloma rapidly or over an extended period after the initial detection of the abnormal monoclonal component. Is MGUS the primary disease? Evidence from the progression of other forms of tumors indicates neoplasms can progress to a malignant state without presenting a benign precursor lesion, and this may occur in myeloma. MGUS nonetheless can represent a step in the plasma cell tumor development. Is MGUS a lesion that should be studied coincidentally with myeloma, rather than focusing on just myeloma alone? This raises the larger question: are there genetic and environmental factors that increase the incidence of MGUS?

The biology of myeloma was discussed in two parts: the clinical disease and the experimental models. There are a number of questions which have not been resolved in the field of clinical myeloma. There has been considerable discussion of whether the entire neoplastic development takes place at the level of the plasma cell or whether antecedent genetic changes begin in the B-cell lineage as far back as the hematopoietic stem cell. It is possible that mutations affecting growth accumulate in a B-cell lineage but only become manifest when the cells begin secreting immunoglobulin. In this context, evidence for expression of inappropriate genes in myeloma was discussed. A second issue concerns the role of IL-6 in myeloma development. IL-6 has been shown to be an important requirement for in vitro growth of myelomas and plasmacytomas; also a few myelomas have been shown to produce IL-6 in an autocrine way. Many, but not all, workers currently consider that IL-6 is generated exogenously by stromal cells, and this raises the question of whether changes in the stromal microenvironment play an important role in plasma cell tumor development. The availability of IL-6 now makes it possible to establish more myeloma lines in culture when appropriate stromal elements are added. Third, myeloma has not thus far been associated with a consistent oncogenic mutation. Interestingly, the c-myc gene has not been activated by chromosomal translocations in clinical myeloma as it is in some of the experimental forms. The general picture that seems to emerge in many of the myeloma cases that have been studied cytogenetically is that there are multiple karyotypic abnormalities, suggesting some genetic instability in these cells. Fourth, the mode of spread of myeloma is not yet clearly established. Bone marrow plasma cells in normal individuals are thought to arise in extramedullary sites as B-lymphocytes that migrate to bone marrow sites. Circulating cells apparently lacking plasma cell morphology have been cultured from the blood with IL-6 and IL-3, and these suggestively could be responsible for sending myeloma cells to different sites.

Three experimental systems were discussed. Most plasmacytomas in mice are induced by the intraperitoneal implantation of plastics or injection of paraffin oils. These agents initiate a complex inflammatory process which appears to be essential for plasmacytoma development as the tumors arise histologically in this abnormal tissue. Plasmacytomagenesis can be inhibited in the BALB/c mouse, a genetically susceptible strain, by treatment with indomethacin; further, plasmacytomas cannot be induced in high incidence in pathogen-free BALB/c mice. These papers emphasize the review of available data, or provide descriptions of ongoing projects and preliminary results. The possibilities for further analyses of collected data are described, and directions for new research on multiple myeloma and related malignancies are suggested. Benign monoclonal gammopathies do arise in mice, particularly the C57BL/KaLwRij mice. In these mice, plasma cell neoplasms resembling multiple myeloma arise spontaneously. The evidence currently suggests that the plasma cell tumors in C57BL/KaLwRij mice do not arise from benign monoclonal gammopathies. Spontaneous plasma cell neoplasms, called immunocytomas, occur in the LOU/C inbred strain of rats. Many of these tumors secrete IgE myeloma proteins. Recently there has been a dramatic and unexplained reduction in the incidence of these tumors in the Louvain colony. Possible factors involved are discussed.

G. IRIS OBRAMS
MICHAEL POTTER

Acknowledgements

We appreciate the key role of the Organ Systems Coordinating Branch, National Cancer Institute, especially Dr. William Straile, in the support and organization of this workshop.

Special recognition is due to Mrs. Edythe Cohen, whose efforts were critical to the editing of the epidemiology manuscripts.

We are especially indebted to Ms. Victoria Rogers, who edited the clinical and experimental manuscripts and compiled this book.

Contents

Monoclonal Gammopathies and Multiple Myeloma

Etiologic Hypotheses

Clinical Studies

Contributors

Descriptive and Analytical Epidemiology

Descriptive Epidemiology of Multiple Myeloma

S.S. Devesa

Epidemiology and Biostatistics Program, Division of Cancer Etiology, National Cancer Institute, Executive Plaza North, Bethesda, MD 20892.

According to estimates by the American Cancer Society, almost 12,000 new cases of multiple myeloma are diagnosed and about 9,000 deaths occur in the United States each year (Silverberg et al, 1990). These account for more than one percent of all cancer cases and almost two percent of deaths due to cancer. Although multiple myeloma may arise at any adult age, it tends to occur in older individuals; the median age at diagnosis was 69.1 years, based on 1973-77 Surveillance, Epidemiology, and End Results (SEER) program data, compared to 65.4 years for all forms of cancer combined (Young et al, 1981).

The impact of this malignancy varies by race and sex (Table 1). Based on data from areas with substantial black populations in the SEER program, incidence rates are more than twice as high among blacks than whites, with the standardized incidence ratio (SIR) being 229 and 239 among men and women, respectively. Whereas rates for many other cancers also are higher among blacks than whites, within the hematopoietic system, multiple myeloma is the only one with a clear excess among blacks. Compared to whites, SIRs range from 88 and 103 for myelocytic leukemia to 67 and 70 for non-Hodgkin's lymphoma, and 66 and 50 for Hodgkin's disease among men and women, respectively. Similar to many other malignancies, a male excess is apparent for multiple myeloma, with rates 39% and 45% higher among men than women among blacks and whites, respectively.

Since the early 1950s, national multiple myeloma mortality rates have more than doubled among whites and about quadrupled among nonwhites (Fig. 1), based on data from the National Center for Health Statistics. Data specific for blacks are available since the early 1970s; their rates are the highest and show the greatest proportional increases. Rates among white men during the early 1980s do not appear to be continuing the prior rate of increase.

The rise in mortality rates occurred predominantly among older age groups (Fig. 2). Among both whites and nonwhites, little change occurred among those under age 50. In the early years, rates increased among most groups over age 50 years, whereas in more recent years the changes have been greatest among those age 70 years and older.

Although multiple myeloma was quite rare in the past, the proportional increase has been one of the largest of any site (Devesa et al 1987), most likely affected by the introduction of improved diagnostic tools over the past several decades (Blattner 1982). Substantial increases in both incidence and mortality have been observed for multiple myeloma in many countries, whereas relatively stable rates have been reported in others (Linos et al 1981, Velez et al 1982, Cuzick et al 1983, Turesson et al 1984, Nandakumar et al 1988, Hansen et al 1989, Cuzick 1990). The variations are believed to be largely the result of differences in diagnostic capability. Striking increases in the older age groups are consistent with improved medical technology and its expanded use in the high-risk older population.

Table 1. Comparison of incidence* of various hematopoietic cancers among blacks and whites in Atlanta, Connecticut, Detroit, and San Francisco-Oakland during 1977-83.

	Males No.	Males Rate	Males SIR#	Females No.	Females Rate	Females SIR#
Multiple myeloma:						
Black	440	10.3	229	424	7.4	239
White	1403	4.5		1411	3.1	
Hodgkin's disease:						
Black	155	2.5	66	95	1.3	50
White	1342	3.8		1027	2.6	
Non-Hodgkin's lymphoma:						
Black	419	8.7	67	363	6.0	70
White	4,202	13.0		4,105	8.6	
Leukemias						
Black	537	11.6	83	451	7.4	93
White	4,310	13.9		3,372	8.0	
Lymphocytic						
Black	229	5.1	88	157	2.6	76
White	1777	5.8		1349	3.4	
Myelocytic						
Black	242	4.9	88	229	3.6	103
White	1762	5.6		1514	3.5	

*Rates per 100,000 person-years, age-adjusted using the 1970 U.S. standard.
#Standardized incidence ratio, relative to the rate among whites in the same geographic areas.
Based on data from the SEER program.

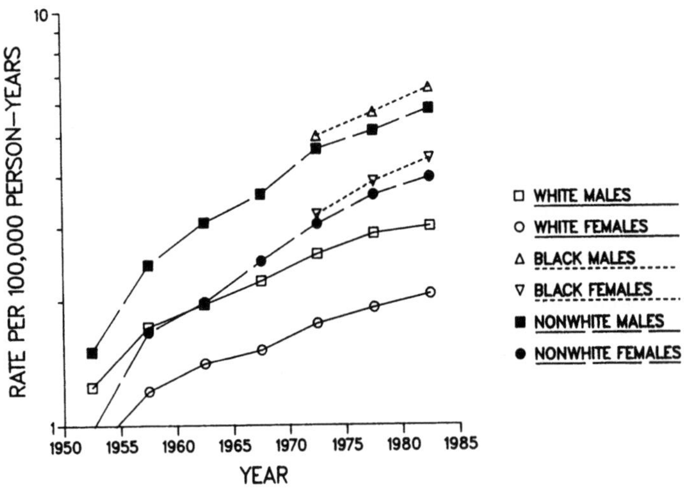

Fig. 1. Age-adjusted (1970) multiple myeloma mortality trends in the US by race and sex, 1950-54--1980-84.

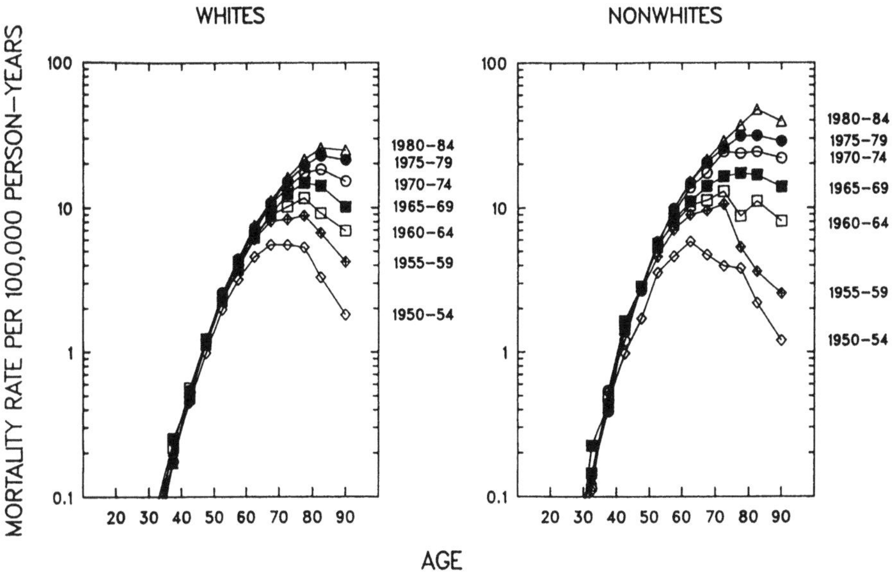

Fig. 2. Age-specific US multiple myeloma mortality curves among whites and nonwhites, 1950-54--1980-84.

During recent years, 1975-85, mortality rates rose consistently with age, except for a slight decline at the oldest ages among blacks (Fig. 3). Among both blacks and whites, the male:female ratio is somewhat smaller at younger than older ages, as indicated by the vertical distance between the curves. On the other hand, the black:white mortality ratio is larger at younger ages; compared to about a 50% excess among the oldest age groups, the ratio approaches three among those under age 50.

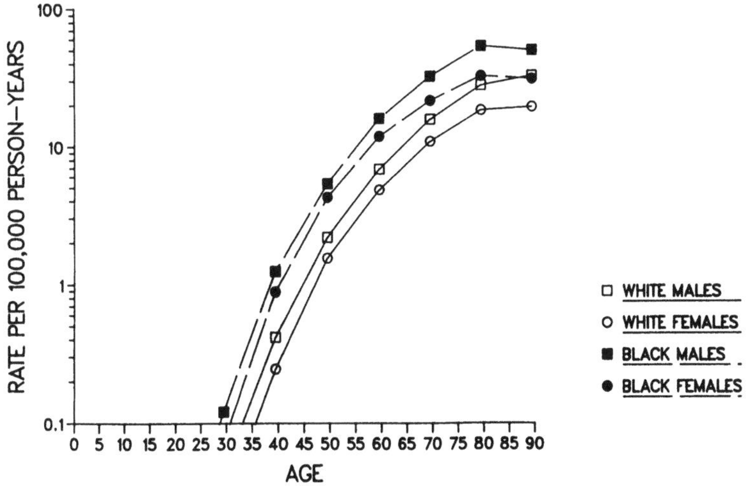

Fig. 3. Age-specific US multiple myeloma mortality rates by race and sex, 1975-85.

In contrast to substantial increases in mortality at the national level, incidence trends since 1969-71 in five areas common to the SEER program, the Third National Cancer Survey (TNCS) (Cutler and Young 1975), and the Connecticut Tumor Registry (Heston et al 1986), indicate that multiple myeloma rates have stabilized among whites since the mid-1970s (Fig. 4) (Devesa et al 1987). Among blacks, increases continued through the 1970s, but rates may have peaked in the early 1980s.

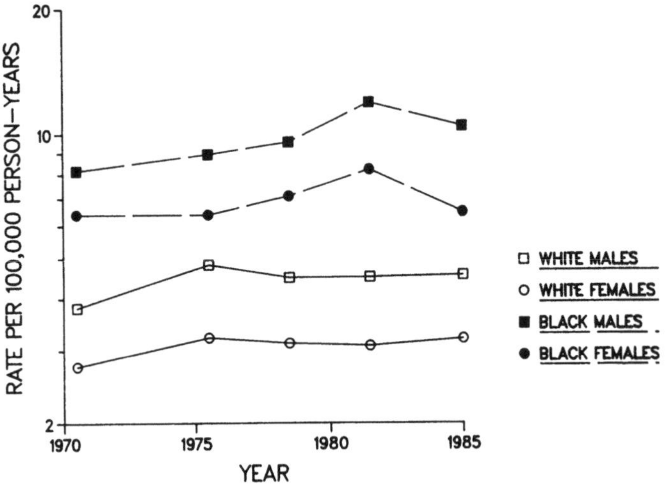

Fig. 4. Trends in age-adjusted (1970) incidence of multiple myeloma in the 5GA by race and sex, 1969-71 to 1984-86.

The age-specific incidence curves are higher than the mortality curves and generally similar in shape (Fig. 5). Although based on somewhat low numbers of cases (32, 37), rates are remarkably similar among black men and women under age 45, but not among whites.

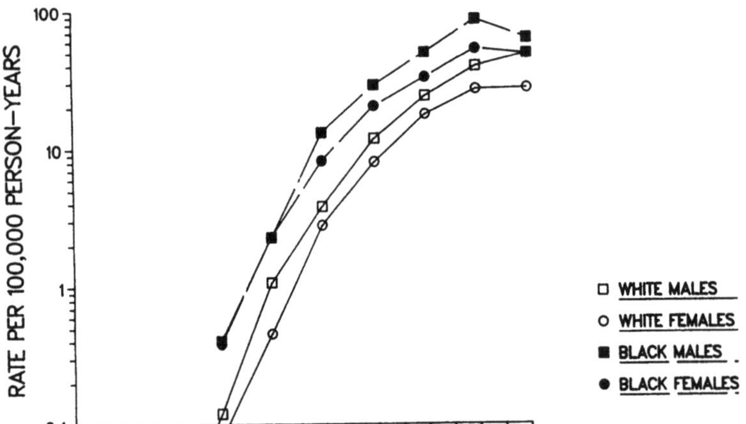

Fig. 5. Age-specific incidence of multiple myeloma in the 5GA by race and sex, 1975-85.

Improvements in relative survival rates occurred during the 1960s and early 1970s, with subsequent increases more modest (Table 2) (National Cancer Institute 1989). Five-year relative survival rates among whites rose from 10-13% to about 25% over the 20-year period. Although data pertaining to blacks during the early years are not available, recent rates indicate that blacks diagnosed with multiple myeloma experience better survival rates than do whites.

Table 2. Five-year relative survival rates (per cent) among patients with multiple myeloma by race and sex, 1960-63 to 1980-85.

	1960-63	1970-73	1974-76	1977-79	1980-85
White males	13	20	22.8	24.2	24.9
White females	10	17	24.9	23.6	26.6
Black males	-	-	28.1	28.3	25.9
Black females	-	-	27.9	36.3	32.0

Data for 1960-73 based on the End Results Group and for 1974-85 based on the SEER program.
Source: National Cancer Institute, 1989.

As seen earlier, considering only those areas with substantial black populations, multiple myeloma incidence rates among blacks are more than twice those among whites (Table 3). Incidence data also are available from the SEER program for several other racial/ethnic groups, although many of the rates are based on somewhat low numbers of cases. Rates

Table 3. Racial/ethnic variation in multiple myeloma incidence* during 1975-85.

	Males			Females		
	No.	Rate	SIR#	No.	Rate	SIR#
In Atlanta, Connecticut, Detroit, San Francisco-Oakland:						
Black	689	10.3	229	623	6.9	223
White	2223	4.5		2217	3.1	
In San Francisco-Oakland and Hawaii:						
Chinese	25	2.3	50	22	1.8	58
Japanese	28	1.7	37	30	1.4	45
Filipino	61	4.7	102	21	2.6	84
White	668	4.6		632	3.1	
In Hawaii:						
Hawaiian	25	6.1	145	27	5.6	224
White	48	4.2		30	2.5	
In New Mexico (and Arizona for American Indians):						
Hispanic	44	2.8	74	50	2.8	104
American Indian	23	3.4	89	31	4.2	156
Anglo	143	3.8		126	2.7	

*Rates per 100,000 person-years, age-adjusted using the 1970 U.S. standard.
#Standardized incidence ratio, relative to the rate among whites in the same geographic areas.
Based on data from the SEER program.

among Asians generally are lower than those among whites living in the same geographic areas, with SIRS of 37 and 45 among Japanese men and women, whereas Hawaiians appear to be at excess risk. Among Hispanics and American Indians, rates among men appear low and among women they are high, relative to whites.

As suggested by the previous table, geographic variation in rates may occur. Although not as notable as for other forms of cancer, regional variation in multiple myeloma mortality has been reported by Pickle et al, with elevated rates in the North Central areas of the United States, particularly among males (Pickle et al 1987). During the early 1950s, myeloma mortality rates were higher in urban than rural areas, but the differences had disappeared by the early 1970s (Greenberg 1983). Among whites in the SEER areas, recent incidence rates among men vary from 5.2 in Seattle to 3.5 in New Mexico, about a 50% difference (Table 4). With the exception of Iowa, where rates are relatively high, myeloma incidence is lower in the states than the cities. Rates among females vary less than 30%, and seven out of nine are in the 3.0-3.2 range.

Table 4. Geographic variation in multiple myeloma incidence rates* among whites, SEER 1975-85.

	MALES		FEMALES	
	No.	Rate	No.	Rate
Seattle	642	5.2	520	3.2
Iowa	821	5.0	754	3.2
Detroit	741	4.8	670	3.2
San Francisco	620	4.6	602	3.1
Atlanta	202	4.4	225	3.2
Connecticut	660	4.2	720	3.1
Utah	218	4.2	196	3.0
Hawaii	48	4.2	30	2.5
New Mexico	187	3.5	176	2.7

*per 100,000 person-years, age-adjusted using the 1970 U.S. standard.
Based on data from the SEER program.

Recent incidence rates vary internationally more than ten-fold, as published in Volume V of <u>Cancer Incidence in Five Continents</u> (Muir et al 1987). Figure 6 shows that rates are highest among blacks in the SEER areas and in Los Angeles, and in Martinique, where the "majority of the population is of African origin, more or less mixed with populations of European origin" (Muir et al, p. 198). Other populations shown representing the Caribbean, Central, and South America have much lower rates and low proportions of blacks. Unfortunately, sub-Saharan Africa was not represented in that Volume. Earlier volumes do not suggest notable excess risks of multiple myeloma among African natives (Waterhouse et al 1976, Waterhouse et al 1982), although case ascertainment may not have been comparable to that in Western countries.

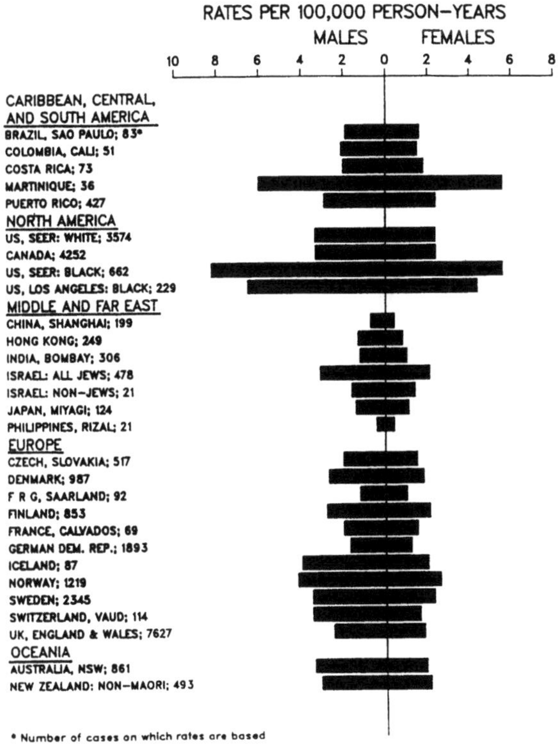

Fig. 6. International variation in age-adjusted (world standard) multiple myeloma incidence rates, approximately 1980.

A comparison of incidence rates among blacks in South Africa and the U.S. indicated similar (elevated) rates (Blattner et al 1979). Rates generally are low in the Middle and Far East, with the exception of Jews in Israel, among whom rates are more comparable to those found in Europe. Within Europe, rates in Scandinavia generally are higher than those in other areas.

Several registries provide rates for urban vs. rural groups (Fig. 7). The largest number of cases come from England and Wales, an area with intermediate rates, where there is no difference in multiple myeloma incidence between urban and rural men, and a slight excess among rural women. In areas with relatively high rates among men, an urban excess is suggested, such as in Norway, Switzerland, and Australia, whereas in areas with lower overall rates, an urban deficit is apparent. That is, there appears to be greater geographic variation in urban than rural rates, particularly among males.

Socioeconomic status has not been uniformly linked to multiple myeloma risk. In the past, positive gradients were suggested, but they may have been diagnostic artifact (Hoover et al 1975, Logan 1982, Johnston et al 1985). Based on data from the TNCS, consistent patterns with income or education are not apparent (Table 5) (Devesa 1979). Modest positive tendencies are suggested among white men, whereas inverse gradients are suggested among white women and black men. None of the trends were

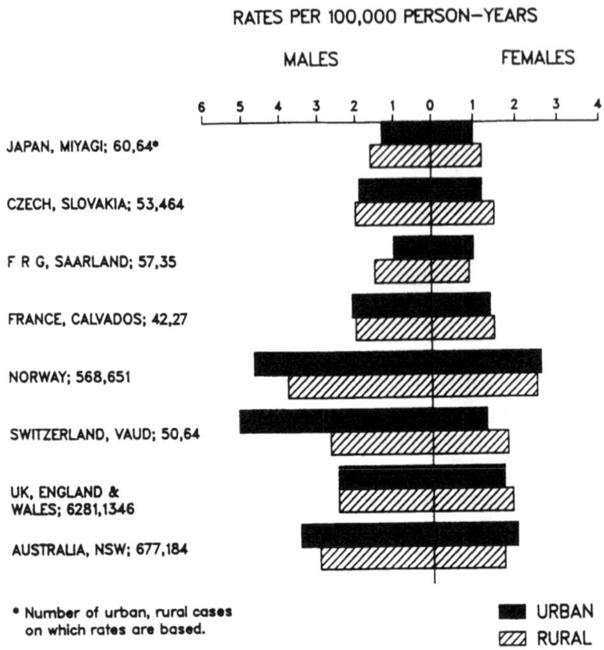

Fig. 7. International urban/rural variation in age-adjusted (world standard) multiple myeloma incidence rates, approximately 1980.

Table 5. Relative risks of multiple myeloma by race, sex, income, and education level, 1969-71.

		Men	Women
Whites: Income:	1 (Low)	.89	1.30
	2	:85	1.42
	3	.88	1.33
	4	.98	1.26
	5 (High)	1.00	1.00
Education:	1 (Low)	.96	1.11
	2	.75	1.10
	3	.95	1.41
	4	.97	1.35
	5 (High)	1.00	1.00
Blacks: Income:	1 (Low)	1.47	1.12
	2	1.36	.89
	3 (High)	1.00	1.00
Education:	1 (Low)	1.24	.89
	2	1.19	1.12
	3 (High)	1.00	1.00

Data from Devesa, 1979.

significant. Adjusting for socioeconomic differences had minimal impact on the black/white incidence ratio (Table 6), which declined slightly among both men and women in the TNCS and among men in the SEER data (Devesa 1979, McWhorter et al 1989). The racial differences in rates remained highly significant, however. Among women in the SEER program, the ratio increased. Socioeconomic factors therefore must play little role in the development of multiple myeloma.

Table 6. Effect of adjustment for socioeconomic status on multiple myeloma black/white incidence ratio.

	Black/white incidence ratio	
	Men	Women
Based on 1969-71 TNCS data (Devesa 1979):		
Adjusted for:		
Age	1.92	1.96
Age, area, income, education	1.67	1.84
Based on 1978-82 SEER data (McWhorter et al 1989):		
Adjusted for:		
Age	2.53	2.30
Age, poverty	2.24	2.37

Thus, we see that the main characteristics of multiple myeloma are its increased frequency at older ages, the excess among blacks and deficits among Asian groups, a possible plateauing of rates with time, inconsistent urban/rural patterns, and little association with socioeconomic status. As survival rates have not changed greatly since the early 1970s, we must look for the means of primary prevention.

I thank Ms. Ruth Parsons of Information Management Services, Inc., for computer and graphics support.

References

Blattner WA (1982) Multiple myeloma and macroglobulinemia. In: Schottenfeld D, Fraumeni JF Jr, eds Cancer epidemiology and prevention. Philadelphia: Saunders 795-813
Blattner WA, Jacobson RJ, Shulman G (1979) Multiple myeloma in South African blacks. Lancet 1979; 1:928-929
Cutler SJ, Young JL Jr, eds (1975) Third national cancer survey: Incidence data. Natl Cancer Inst Monogr 41:1-454
Cuzick J, Velez R, Doll R (1983) International variations and temporal trends in mortality from multiple myeloma. Int J Cancer 32:13-19
Cuzick J (1990) International time trends for multiple myeloma. (In Press)
Devesa SS (1979) The association of cancer incidence with income and education. Ph.D. dissertation, Johns Hopkins University
Devesa SS, Silverman DT, Young JL Jr, et al (1987) Cancer incidence and mortality trends among whites in the United States, 1947-84. JNCI 79:701-770
Greenberg MR (1983) Urbanization and cancer mortality: The United States experience, 1950-1975. Monographs in epidemiology and biostatistics, Volume 4. New York: Oxford University Press
Hansen NE, Karle H, Olsen JH (1989) Trends in the incidence of multiple myeloma in Denmark 1943-1982: A study of 5500 patients. Eur J Haematol 42:72-76

Heston JF, Kelly JB, Meigs JW, et al, eds (1986) Forty-five years of cancer incidence in Connecticut: 1935-79. Natl Cancer Inst Monogr 70:1-706
Hoover R, Mason TJ, McKay FW, et al (1975) Geographic patterns of cancer mortality in the United States. In: Fraumeni JF Jr (ed): Persons at High Risk of Cancer- An Approach to Cancer Etiology and Control. Academic Press, Inc, New York, pp 343-360
Johnston JM, Grufferman S, Bourguet CC, et al (1985) Socioeconomic status and risk of multiple myeloma. J Epidemiol Comm Health 39:175-178
Linos A, Kyle RA, O'Fallon WM, et al (1981) Incidence and secular trend of multiple myeloma in Olmstead County, Minnesota: 1965-77. JNCI 66:17-20
Logan WPD (1982) Cancer mortality by occupation and social class, 1851-1971. IARC Scientific Publications No 36. Lyon: IARC
McWhorter WP, Schatzkin AG, Horm JW, et al (1989) Contribution of socioeconomic status to black/white differences in cancer incidence. Cancer 63:982-987
Muir C, Waterhouse J, Mack T, et al (eds) (1987) Cancer incidence in five continents, Volume V. IARC Scientific Publication No 88. Lyon: International Agency for Research on Cancer
Nandakumar A, English DR, Dougan LE, Armstrong BK (1988) Incidence and outcome of multiple myeloma in Western Australia, 1960-1984. Aust NZ J Med 18:774-779
National Cancer Institute (1989) Annual cancer statistics review, 1988, including a report on the status of cancer control. Bethesda, MD: NCI
Pickle LW, Mason TJ, Howard N, et al (1987) Atlas of U.S. cancer mortality among whites: 1950-1980. Washington, DC: US Govt Printing Office, DHHS Publication No (NIH) 87-2900
Silverberg E, Boring CC, Squires TS (1990) Cancer statistics, 1990. CA-A Cancer Journal for Clinicians 40:9-26
Turesson I, Zettervall O, Cuzick J, et al (1984) Comparison of trends in the incidence of multiple myeloma in Malmo, Sweden, and other countries, 1950-1979. N Engl J Med 310:421-424
Velez R, Beral V, Cuzick J (1982) Increasing trends of multiple myeloma mortality in England and Wales; 1950-79: Are the changes real? JNCI 69:387-392
Waterhouse J, Muir C, Correa P, et al (eds) (1976) Cancer incidence in five continents, Volume III. IARC Scientific Publication No 15. Lyon: International Agency for Research on Cancer
Waterhouse J, Muir C, Shanmugaratnam K, et al (eds) (1982) Cancer incidence in five continents, Volume IV. IARC Scientific Publication No. 42. Lyon: International Agency for Research on Cancer
Young JL Jr, Percy CL, Asire AJ, eds (1981) Surveillance, epidemiology, end results: Incidence and mortality data, 1973-77. Natl Cancer Inst Monogr 57:1-1082

Epidemiologic Studies of Multiple Myeloma: Occupation and Radiation Effects

D.A. Riedel

Environmental Epidemiology Branch, National Cancer Institute, NIH, Executive Plaza North, Suite 418, Bethesda, MD 20892

INTRODUCTION

The focus of this summary is a review of the more recent multiple myeloma epidemiologic studies that address occupation and radiation exposures. Most of the investigations have been conducted in white populations, with few focusing on blacks alone, or factors that might explain the black/white differences in risk of this cancer.

Agricultural occupations are of considerable interest due to the large number of studies and associations that exist. Within agriculture, studies have focused on type of farming including crops or livestock, and chemical exposures. Agricultural chemicals frequently considered include fertilizers and pesticides.

The second major area of investigation includes occupations in non-agricultural settings covering a variety of exposures. Some exposures are better described than others. In many studies, myeloma has been associated with certain industries, but the actual job exposure was not given in any detail. Associations have been reported with specific types of substances such as 1) benzene, and 2) with employment in various industries including metal, petroleum refining and products, rubber manufacturing, and leather, wood, and textiles.

Under radiation, the third major area of investigation, there are three major categories of exposure: incidental or environmental exposure (such as atomic bomb survivors or residents near nuclear facilities), exposure to diagnostic and therapeutic medical X-rays, and occupational exposure. Several occupational groups linked to radiation, including radiologists, radium dial workers, and nuclear workers, have an increased occurrence of multiple myeloma.

RESULTS

Of all the occupations, agriculture has the most consistent association with myeloma risk. Out of 19 studies published between 1978 and 1989, there were 28 positive associations between agriculture and risk for multiple myeloma (Table 1). Only three studies reviewed did not show an association with agriculture (not shown). Twenty-five of the positive associations were statistically significant. The majority of these reports provided risks associated with farming as an occupation rather than with specific exposures. Five studies noted excesses among livestock farmers, and four studies noted associations with use of pesticides and fertilizers. Only one study of farming exposures included blacks who were found to have a significant increase in risk.

Table 1. Multiple myeloma agriculture literature. Positive studies published between 1978 and 1989.

Exposure	No. Associations	Risk Range
Farming	18	1.2 - 3.4
Farm Animals	5	1.3 - 2.0
Pesticides/ Fertilizers	4	1.7 - 4.3
Grain	1	2.4
TOTAL	28	1.2 - 4.3

Among 34 studies of non-agricultural occupations, there were 42 positive associations (Table 2). The miscellaneous category had the highest number of positive associations and included exposure to asbestos, chemicals, paints, and dusts among workers in various industries in addition to hairdressers, and chimney sweeps. Work in the metal industry had the second highest number of positive associations, followed by petroleum and rubber manufacturing industries. Exposures incurred in wood and pulp industries may be due to the chemicals used in processing or to wood dust. One study of metal exposure noted a significant association among nonwhites.

Table 2. Multiple myeloma occupation literature. Positive studies published between 1976 and 1989.

Exposure	No. Associations	Risk Range
Miscellaneous	15	1.1 - 6.2
Metals	9	1.1 - 2.5
Petroleum	6	1.2 - 3.7
Rubber Manufacturing	5	1.3 - 4.5
Leather	3	1.9 - 3.5
Wood	2	1.8 - 3.2
Textile	1	2.7
Benzene	1	4.1
TOTAL	42	1.1 - 6.2

Radiation is biologically plausible as a risk exposure for multiple myeloma since previous associations have been observed for leukemia and radiation. However, there are differences in types of radiation and exposure. Black/white differences were not addressed in any of the radiation studies.

Among studies of multiple myeloma and radiation (Table 3), the most consistent risk has occurred among the atomic bomb survivors. While there are a large number of associations for medical X-rays and residents near nuclear facilities, none of them were significant and many had a risk below 1.0 (the null value). Two associations were significant for multiple myeloma risk among nuclear facility workers, although the workers' exact exposures were not well described. There was a significant risk among radium dial workers who incurred their radium exposures either internally or externally.

Table 3. Multiple myeloma radiation literature. All studies published between 1981 and 1989.

Exposure	No. Associations	Risk Range
Atomic Bomb Survivors	3	1.0 - 3.2
Diag. X-Ray Workers	1	0.0
Medical X-Rays	7	0.9 - 2.9
Nuclear Facility		
Workers	4	0.8 - 14.7
Residents	5	0.8 - 2.7
Radium Dial Workers	1	2.3
TOTAL	21	0.0 - 14.7

DISCUSSION

When interpreting the associations between multiple myeloma and occupation and radiation, several issues must be considered. Definitions of exposures differ from study to study. It is difficult to draw conclusions between the individual associations and multiple myeloma risk from analyses which incorporate broad versus specific exposure categories. For example, most investigations of non-agricultural exposures have been based on occupation/industry categories, or job title. This creates a problem of interpretation because specific exposures are not identified, and actual exposures vary by industry with regard to the same job title.

There may be problems regarding the diagnosis of multiple myeloma, particularly in mortality studies. In the evaluation of mortality within occupation or industry cohorts using ICD codes, code 203--the code for death from multiple myeloma, is frequently skipped or lumped with other hematopoietic malignancies.

Agriculture and radiation exposures have been linked with an increased risk for multiple myeloma. The agriculture association has been seen in a number of different countries including Sweden, the U.K., the U.S., Canada, Australia, and New Zealand. Pesticides have been linked with other hematopoietic and lymphatic cancers, thus increasing the biologic plausibility for the association with multiple myeloma.

Associations of myeloma and other non-agricultural exposures have been noted, but information regarding dose-response, strength of association, specificity of association, and replication of results by different studies is not consistent. Possible explanations for the lack of consistency may include difficulties in isolating the precise exposure under study in a population from other competing exposures, the small number of exposed cases, and that the associations observed may be chance occurrences.

Several studies have found associations between prior radiation exposure and multiple myeloma. The most consistent associations for radiation have been observed among atomic bomb survivors who experienced high instantaneous doses of radiation, and among radiologists and radium dial workers who received lower doses over a long period of time. Radiation has been linked with some lymphatic and hematopoietic cancers including acute and myeloid leukemias, and non-Hodgkin's lymphoma, but not with chronic lymphocytic leukemia.

In conclusion, there are very few epidemiologic studies that consider blacks separately, and none which discuss black/white differences for risk of multiple myeloma. Future studies should include better definition of exposure in an attempt to explain differences in risk for multiple myeloma among blacks and whites.

REFERENCE

Riedel DA, Pottern LM, Blattner WA (1990) The epidemiology of multiple myeloma. In: Wiernik PH, Canellos GP, Kyle RA, Schiffer CA (eds) Neoplastic diseases of the blood, 2nd edn. Churchill Livingstone, New York, in press

SUGGESTED READING

Boffetta P, Stellman SD, Garfinkel L (1989) A case-control study of multiple myeloma nested in the American Cancer Society prospective study. Int J Cancer 43:554-559

Burmeister LF, Everett GD, Van Lier SF, Isacson P (1983) Selected cancer mortality and farm practices in Iowa. Am J Epidemiol 118:72-77

Cuzick J, De Stavola B (1988) Multiple myeloma - a case-control study. Br J Cancer 57:516-520

Delzell E, Grufferman S (1985) Mortality among white and nonwhite farmers in North Carolina, 1976-1978. Am J Epidemiol 121:391-402

Flodin U, Frederiksson M, Persson B (1987) Multiple myeloma and engine exhausts, fresh wood, and creosote: a case-referent study. Am J Ind Med 12:519-529

Ichimaru M, Ishimaru T, Mikami M, et al. (1982) Multiple myeloma among atomic bomb survivors in Hiroshima and Nagasaki, 1950-1976: relationship to radiation dose absorbed by marrow. J Natl Cancer Inst 69:323-328

Linet MS, Harlow SD, McLaughlin JK (1987) A case-control study of multiple myeloma in whites: chronic antigenic stimulation, occupation, and drug use. Cancer Res 47:2978-2981

Matanoski GM, Seltser R, Sartwell PE, et al. (1975) The current mortality rates of radiologists and other physician specialists: specific causes of death. Am J Epidemiol 101:199-210

Morris PD, Koepsell TD, Daling JR, et al. (1986) Toxic substance exposure and multiple myeloma: a case-control study. J Natl Cancer Inst 76:987-994

Multiple Myeloma in Iowa Farmers

Leon F. Burmeister

Department of Preventive Medicine and Environmental Health, University of Iowa, Iowa City, Iowa 52242

INTRODUCTION

Milham first reported significantly increased mortality in farmers from multiple myeloma in a study completed in Washington state based on deaths from 1950-1971 (1). Some years later, Cantor and Blair reported similar results in Wisconsin farmers (2). Male deaths from 1968-1976 were studied, resulting in an odds ratio of 1.4 for mortality from multiple myeloma in farmers. The highest odds ratio (OR) was reported for decedents over 65 (OR = 1.5). The ORs were significantly elevated in the 15 counties with high chicken inventory (OR = 1.6), high fertilizer usage (OR = 1.7), and high insecticide usage (OR = 1.9). The odds ratios in the remaining counties were not significantly elevated for these production and usage characteristics.

Other studies describing multiple myeloma in farmers have been summarized by Blair et al. (3). In addition to the Washington and Wisconsin studies, multiple myeloma has been associated with farming in Oregon (4) and Texas (5). In New Zealand, multiple myeloma was greater in farmers less than 65 (6); however, there was no apparent association for crop or livestock farmers in New Zealand.

IOWA STUDIES

Mortality from multiple myeloma was significantly increased in white male Iowa farmers during the period 1971-1978 (7). The overall proportionate mortality ratio was 1.27; however, the proportionate morality ratio for Iowa farmers less than 65 was 1.71.

Case-control analyses of death certificate data in Iowa from 1964-1978 indicated a significant odds ratio for mortality from multiple myeloma in white male Iowa farmers of 1.48 (8). The odds ratios were significantly elevated only for those born after 1890, indicating that modern farming practices (post World War II) might be associated with multiple myeloma mortality. Aggregate analyses based on county crop and livestock production indicated that herbicide usage, insecticide usage, and production of egg-laying chickens were associated with mortality from multiple myeloma in the highest 33 counties for usage or production, but not in the remaining 66 counties. This was true for those born from 1890-1900, as well as the cohort born after 1900. There were no significant associations for those born before 1890.

A recent study of death certificates in Iowa has indicated that mortality from multiple myeloma in farmers has decreased for the period 1979-1986 (9). The PMR for farmers under 65 was 0.88 and, for those 65 or older, the PMR was 0.96.

Risk factors not associated with farming have also been suggested for multiple myeloma (10). These include exposure to ionizing radiation; previous immunosuppressive diseases; occupational exposure to lead, arsenic, and asbestos; manufacture of plastics, wood products, leather products, rubber products, and petrochemical products; sibling history of multiple myeloma; and diseases such as scleroderma, rheumatoid arthritis, and chronic dermatitis.

Because of the many inherent methodologic deficiencies of death certificate studies and the lack of individual risk factor assessment, a case-control study was completed using incident cases within a defined geographic region with a high proportion of farmers.

Pathologically confirmed cases of multiple myeloma diagnosed from January, 1982 through March, 1984 were identified by the State Health Registry of Iowa. Controls for live cases diagnosed in 1984 were selected by random digit dialing. Controls for deceased cases diagnosed in 1984 were matched for sex, 5 year age group, and year of death and were selected from the 1984 death certificate tape provided by the Iowa State Health Department. Controls included 130 persons from the simultaneously completed collaborative case-control study of Iowa and Minnesota males diagnosed with leukemia and non-Hodgkin's lymphoma, supplemented by 38 living and 7 deceased subjects matched to 1984 cases. The previously interviewed controls were matched to multiple myeloma cases identified in 1982 and 1983. They also were matched by sex, age group, and vital status. Deceased controls were further matched by year of death.

The number of cases initially identified as eligible was 235. Only 198 of these cases were actually interviewed because of physician refusal to allow interview (4), unable to locate (8), and respondent refusal (25). All cases for whom an interview was completed also had pathology review to confirm their diagnosis. Adequate information for diagnostic confirmation was available on 175 cases on whom analyses were completed. Further details of the study, such as questionnaire verification and pathology procedures, are described elsewhere (11).

Multiple logistic regression based on a one-to-one matching of cases and controls was utilized to evaluate suggested risk factors. The results for selected agricultural risk factors are summarized in Table 1. The only risk factor that achieved statistical significance is the handling of insecticides. It must be emphasized that the latter risk factor combines the handling of insecticides in agricultural settings and nonagricultural settings, such as home gardening.

Odds ratios for exposures to classes of herbicides, crop insecticides, and livestock insecticides are summarized in Tables 2-4. These odds ratios are generally larger than one; however, none are statistically significant. It appears that the livestock insecticides have caused lower odds ratios for multiple myeloma incidence than both the insecticides and herbicides used on crops.

Table 1. Estimated Odds Ratios for Incidence of Multiple Myeloma in Iowa Males, 1982 through March, 1984, for Selected Agricultural Exposures

Risk Factor	Odds Ratio
Ever worked on a farm	1.00
Applied herbicides	1.11
Applied insecticides	1.79[1]
Applied garden herbicides	1.28
Applied crop herbicides	1.12
Applied garden insecticides	1.38
Applied crop insecticides	1.50
Applied livestock insecticides	1.34
Exposure to gasoline, kerosene, or diesel fuel	1.29
Acre-years of corn	1.04
Acre-years of soybeans	1.02
Poultry years	1.01

[1] $p < .05$

Table 2. Estimated Odds Ratios for Incidence of Multiple Myeloma in Iowa Males, 1982 through March, 1984, for Herbicide Exposure

Class	Odds Ratio
Amides	1.40
Benzoics	1.22
Bipyridiliums	1.00
Diazine	1.29
Dinitroanilines	2.00
Phenoxy	1.04
Thiocarbamates	2.25
Triazine	1.29
Ureas	2.00
Unclass., other	2.00

Table 3. Estimated Odds Ratios for Incidence of Multiple Myeloma in Iowa Males, 1982 through March, 1984, for Crop Insecticide Exposure

Class	Odds Ratio
Organochlorines	1.53
Organophosphates	1.31
Carbamates	1.83
Arsenicals	0.50
Others	1.20

Table 4. Estimated Odds Ratios for Incidence of Multiple Myeloma in Iowa Males, 1982 through March, 1984, for Livestock Insecticide Exposures

Class	Odds Ratio
Organochlorines	1.44
Organophosphates	1.22
Carbamates	1.00
Nicotine	1.20
Pyrethrins	1.00
Flyspray, NOS[1]	1.52
NOS	0.57

[1] NOS means not otherwise specified

Nonagricultural risk factors are summarized in Table 5. Previous sinus and bone infections appear as possible risk factors. The next highest odds ratio is for use of hair dye; however, it is not statistically significant.

Table 5. Estimated Odds Ratios for Incidence of Multiple Myeloma in Iowa Males, 1982 through March, 1984, for Selected Nonagricultural Exposures

Risk Factor	Odds Ratio
Any radiation exposure	1.00
Handle radioactive materials	0.33
Use of tobacco	1.06
Handle asbestos	0.90
Cancer in relatives	1.28
Previous rheumatoid arthritis	0.83
Cats kept indoors	1.21
Drink beer weekly	1.29
Drink liquor weekly	1.44
Use unpasteurized cream	1.39
Use any unpasteurized product	1.50
Exposure to benzene	0.67
Exposure to hair dyes	2.67
Previous sinus infections	3.25[1]
Previous bone infections	7.39[1]

[1] $p < .05$

DISCUSSION

Most of the suspected agricultural risk factors previously implicated by mortality studies of multiple myeloma in farmers were not statistically significant in the Iowa case-control study. An important consideration is the possibility that multiple myeloma is becoming less important in Iowa as indicated by PMRs less than one for the years 1979-1986. An additional indication of changing mortality rates from multiple myeloma is given in the atlas of cancer mortality (12). The north-central Iowa region has been identified as a concern by the atlas for the period 1950-1978, with the strongest decade of concern being 1960-69. This area remained significantly high in the 1970's, but in the 1960's it was significantly high as well as being in the highest 10% nationally.

In a previous Iowa study (8), one of the agricultural practices most consistently associated with mortality from multiple myeloma was the raising of egg-laying chickens. That study cited a potential link of Marek's disease, a herpes virus-induced malignant lymphoma in chickens, with reticuloendothelial neoplasms in humans. It was also noted (8) that poultry farming has drastically declined in Iowa in recent years and that mortality from human reticuloendothelial cancers might very well decrease. This study supports that conjecture as does the fact that leukemia no longer has significantly elevated PMRs from 1979-1986 in Iowa.

However, this study does indicate continued concern with the handling of pesticides, especially crop insecticides and herbicides. Although there was not sufficient power to detect risk factors that were not prevalent among farmers, such as handling specific classes of insecticides and herbicides, these odds ratios were consistently above 1.0. Consequently, careful handling and application of pesticides continues to be a recommended practice for farmers.

REFERENCES

Milham S Jr. Occupational mortality in Washington State, 1950-1971. Vol 1. Rockville, MD: NIOSH, 1976 [DHEW publication No. (NIH) 76-175-A].

Cantor KP and Blair A. Farming and mortality from multiple myeloma: A case-control study with the use of death certificates. JNCI 1984; 72:251-255.

Blair A, Malkar H, Cantor KP, Burmeister LF, and Wiklund K. Cancer among farmers: A review. Scand J Work Environ Health 1985;11:397-407.

Milham S. Leukemia and multiple myeloma in farmers. Am J Epidemiol 1971; 94:307-310.

Agu AU, Christensen BL, and Buffler PA. Geographical patterns of multiple myeloma: Racial and industrial correlates, state of Texas, 1969-71. JNCI 1980; 65:735-738.

Pearce N, Smith A, and Fisher D. Malignant lymphoma and multiple myeloma linked with agricultural occupations in New Zealand cancer registry-based study. Am J Epidemiol 1985; 121:225-237.

Burmeister LF. Cancer mortality in Iowa farmers, 1971-1978. JNCI 1981; 66:461-4.

Burmeister LF, Everett GD, Van Lier SF, and Isacson P. Selected cancer mortality and farm practices in Iowa. Am J Epidemiol 1983;118:72-77.

Burmeister LF. Cancer in Iowa farmers: recent results. American Journal of Industrial Medicine (in press).

Blattner WA. Epidemiology of multiple myeloma and related plasma cell disorders: An analytic review. 1980, Elsevier North Holland, Inc.

Burmeister LF. A case-control study of multiple myeloma in Iowa men (submitted for publication).

Atlas of U.S. Cancer Mortality Among Whites: 1950-1980. U.S. Government Printing Office, Washington, D.C.

Risk of Multiple Myeloma, Allergies and Agricultural Exposures

Gallagher, Richard P.
Skippen, Diane H.

Division of Epidemiology, Biometry and Occupational Oncology, British Columbia Cancer Agency, 600 West 10th Avenue, Vancouver, B.C., Canada V6M 2L1

INTRODUCTION

A number of studies conducted recently have suggested that farmers are at elevated risk of multiple myeloma (Cantor and Blair 1984, Burmeister et al 1983, Boffetta et al 1989). We have conducted a small case-control study of multiple myeloma in the province of British Columbia in order to investigate the influence of medical history, smoking, alcohol consumption, occupation, some aspects of diet, and other factors on risk of the disease. This paper summarizes the results.

METHODS

A group of 84 myeloma patients was included in this study comprising 49 males and 35 females. To maximize the patient numbers for interview, we elected to include all surviving myeloma patients (prevalent cases) seen at the Vancouver Clinic of the BC Cancer Agency during the years 1972-1978 (32 patients), as well as the 52 cases referred to the Vancouver Clinic from 1979-1981 (incident cases).

All patients not included in the study had died prior to our request for interview. No cases refused participation.

Two control groups were selected. The first consisted of 84 Vancouver Clinic patients with head and neck tumours and the second group included a variety of tumours including digestive system (26 patients), cutaneous basal cell carcinoma (10), breast and female genital (27), male genital (7), hematopoietic (13), and brain (1). All controls had been treated between 1977 and 1980, and were matched to cases by sex, within 5 year age groups, and by year of diagnosis within 5 years.

Both cases and controls were interviewed by trained interviewer using a standard questionnaire. A total of 119 variables were covered during the course of each interview and special emphasis was placed on occupation and presence of prior autoimmune disease. As this study was meant to be an initial overview of possible etiologic factors, relatively little detail was collected on individual variables.

Data were analyzed using initially univariate methods to evaluate odds ratios. Finally, a conditional logistic regression model for matched data sets was applied (Breslow & Day, 1980).

RESULTS

Initial comparisons of cases and controls revealed that marital status and educational levels of the case group were similar to those of the non-head and neck control group. The head and neck control group appeared to have a somewhat lower educational attainment level, perhaps indicating a reduced socio-economic status level by comparison with both cases and non-head and neck controls.

For most analyses, the two control groups were combined, giving two controls per patient. However, for factors known to be affected by socio-economic status such as tobacco and alcohol use, only the non head and neck control group was used.

Myeloma patients reported more prior allergies than controls as shown in Table 1. A greater proportion of cases than controls reported prior treatment for allergies, including special diets, drugs and injections. The character of the allergies demonstrated also appeared to differ between cases and controls, with nearly one-half the symptoms reported by controls as being breathing difficulties while less than 20% of myeloma patients with allergies reported this symptom. Myeloma patients described primarily skin rashes, swellings and hives but more specific data on symptoms was not available.

No difference was seen between prevalence and incident cases in proportions reporting allergies. No association was seen between risk of myeloma and presence of a variety of autoimmune diseases including systemic lupus erythematosus, rheumatoid arthritis or ankylosing spondylitis.

Information on occupational background was collected in two ways. Each respondent completed a checklist of occupations and industries common to British Columbia and additionally more detailed data was collected on each job the respondent had held for one or more years. Analysis of the detailed occupational data revealed an elevated risk of myeloma in individuals who were employed in farming occupations (Table 2), however no increasing risk with increasing duration of work was seen. The association was most pronounced in the incident myeloma cases, with a much weaker association seen among the prevalent myeloma case group. Unfortunately no further data on the type of farming the respondents were engaged in was collected.

Exposure to processed grain, as recorded on the occupational checklist, showed a non-significant increased odds ratio. Since work with grain is dusty, we created an index of dust exposure for each occupation in the data file and applied this to the detailed occupational data. When exposures were cumulated, myeloma patients appear to have greater exposure to dusty workplace conditions than did controls; however, this association disappeared when farming as an occupation was removed from the analysis. No further associations were detected between myeloma and other dusts, including asbestos, metal and textile, or wood dusts, coal or silica.

No significant differences between cases and non-head and neck controls were seen for smoking or alcohol consumption. No association was seen with occupational exposure to ionizing radiation, possibly because there is virtually no nuclear industry in British Columbia.

An examination of dietary factors showed no association with meats, fish, tea, coffee or spicy foods, as measured by food consumption frequency data.

DISCUSSION

Long term survival is poor for multiple myeloma, and the fact that only 20% of total cases referred to the Vancouver Clinic over the years 1972-1981 were interviewed raises the possibility that associations detected in this study may be due to selection bias.

Since the 32 prevalent cases diagnosed from 1972-1978 had survived to be interviewed, it seems likely that their disease was less severe or that they had a better response to treatment than cases who had died. Although the odds ratios for allergies and allergy treatment were similar comparing incident and prevalent cases, the association with farming was seen predominantly in the incident case group. Bearing in mind that this study examined a total of 119 variables, it is also possible that some of our significant findings may be due to chance.

Despite such potential drawbacks, however, it would appear that the study findings are in accord with several U.S. studies showing elevated risk in farmers (Cantor & Blair 1984, Burmeister et al 1983, Milham 1971).

Two of these studies showed that farmers in working in countries with heavy insecticide and herbicide use or with large chicken populations were at highest risk (Cantor & Blair 1984, Burmeister et al 1983). No details about the type of farming done were available on the subjects interviewed for our study.

The increased risk of myeloma in subjects with prior allergies is of interest because of other reports in the literature of myeloma in allergy sufferers (Pearce et al 1986, Linet et al 1987). Finally, it should be emphasized that the largest study conducted to date (Koepsell et al 1987) has not confirmed our findings, and until more evidence emerges, they must be used with caution.

Table 1. Allergies and Multiple Myeloma

Exposure	Myeloma Cases No. (%)	Myeloma Controls No. (%)	O.R.*	p value	95% C.I.
Prior allergies	24 (28.6)	19 (11.3)	3.1	<.001	1.6,6.3
Prior treatment for allergies	11 (13.1)	7 (4.2)	3.5	0.02	1.1,10.6

*O.R. - Odds ratio

Table 2. Farming and Multiple Myeloma

Exposure	Myeloma Cases No. (%)	Myeloma Controls No. (%)	O.R.*	p value	95% C.I.
Farm worker	31 (36.9)	38 (22.6)	2.2	.01	1.2,4.0
Exposure to processed grain	9 (10.7)	8 (4.8)	2.4	.09	0.9,6.6
Work in industry conditions	38 (45.2)	45 (32.1)	2.1	.02	1.1,4.0

*O.R. = odds ratio

REFERENCES

Cantor KP, Blair A (1984) Farming and mortality from multiple myeloma: a case-control study with the use of death certificates. J Natl Cancer Inst 72:251-255.
Burmeister LF, Everett GD, Vanhier SF, Isaacson P (1983) Selected cancer mortality and farm practises in Iowa. Am J Epidemiol 188:72-77.
Boffetta P, Stellman SD, Garfinkel L (1989) A case-control study of multiple myeloma vested in the American Cancer Society prospective study. Int J Cancer 43:554-559.
Breslow NE, Day NE (1980) Statistical Methods in Cancer Research Vol I. IARC Scientific Publication #32, International Agency for Research on Cancer, Lyon.
Milham JS (1971) Leukemia and multiple myeloma in farmers. Am J Epidemiol 94:307-310.
Pearce NE, Smith AH, Howard JK et al (1986). Case-control study of multiple myeloma and farming. Br J Cancer 54:493-500.
Linet MS, Harlow SD, McLaughlin JK (1987). A case-control study of multiple myeloma in whites: chronic antigenic stimulation, occupation and drug use. Cancer Res 47:2978-2981.
Koepsell TD, Daling JR, Weiss NS et al (1987) Antigenic stimulation and the occurrence of multiple myeloma. Am J Epidemiol 126:1051-1062.

Leads for Future Studies from a Case-Control Study of Occupational Exposures and Multiple Myeloma in Denmark

E.F. Heineman[1], J. Olsen[2], L.M. Pottern[1], M.R. Gomez[1], E. Raffn[2], and A. Blair[1]

[1]Occupational Studies Section, Environmental Epidemiology Branch, National Cancer Institute, Rockville, Maryland, U.S.A.
[2]Danish Cancer Registry, Copenhagen, Denmark

INTRODUCTION

Although multiple myeloma is not considered an occupational cancer, it has been linked with a number of occupations and occupational exposures (Riedel 1990). The existence in Denmark of a national cancer registry and the availability of employment records on a national level presented a unique opportunity to explore further the role of occupation in multiple myeloma. A collaborative population-based case-control study of multiple myeloma was conducted by the National Cancer Institute and the Danish Cancer Registry to refine and develop hypotheses regarding occupational exposures in the origin of multiple myeloma. The incidence of multiple myeloma among men in Denmark (2.7 per 100,000 in 1977-82) is similar to that in Finland, the United Kingdom, and among U.S. white men, suggesting that clues generated from this investigation may be relevant to many countries. A manuscript currently in preparation will describe results for the males in detail. This paper presents two preliminary findings, however, in the hope that they may be of value to other investigators.

METHODS

Briefly, cases of multiple myeloma were those newly diagnosed in Denmark between 1970 and 1984 and reported to the Danish Cancer Registry. Ninety-two percent had been verified histologically. Controls, matched 4:1 to cases on age, sex, and calendar-year were selected from the Central Population Registry, which lists all Danish citizens, for the year in which the cases were diagnosed. Subjects were excluded if they were diagnosed with a prior malignancy more than three months before the diagnosis of the case; if they were less than 18 years old; or if their year of birth was before 1897. Information on industries in which subjects were employed was obtained from the Supplementary Pension Fund, which since 1964 has recorded all employments of Danish citizens aged 16-66. Occupation was the last job title reported on subjects' tax records. For each industry-occupation combination, Danish industrial hygienists evaluated the likelihood of exposure to 47 substances suggested to be associated with multiple myeloma by a review of the literature. Men included in the analyses were the 1098 (90% of) cases and 4169 (85% of) controls with information available on occupation or at least one industry.

RESULTS AND DISCUSSION

In this study, multiple myeloma was associated with exposure to gasoline and to engine exhaust. The effects of the two exposures could not be disentangled. A previous study has reported elevated risks of myeloma among men likely to be exposed to engine exhaust (Flodin 1987). Additional studies to further evaluate these apparent associations are needed. Of particular value would be inclusion of biologic measures of exposure to gasoline and engine exhausts. Depending on the design of such a study, levels of lead in blood measured around the time of likely exposure could serve as markers of past exposure to engine exhaust. Confounding by occupational and non-occupational sources of lead exposure, such as ingestion of leaded paint, for example, would need to be considered. Although lead exposure itself has been suggested as a potential risk factor for myeloma (Greene 1979), this study provided no evidence of such an association.

In these Danish men, multiple myeloma was also associated with exposure to phthalates, a class of plasticizers widely used in plastics, paints, rubber, and other products. This finding is consistent with those of previous studies which found excesses of myeloma among paint manufacturing workers (Lundberg 1986), rubber workers (Delzell 1985; Monson 1976), and food processing workers, particularly butchers (Cuzick 1988) and with exposure to paint-related products (Morris 1986), and plastics (Morris 1986). Risk increased with both duration and probability of exposure to phthalates, rising to 2.5 (95% CI=0.9-7.0) among men judged to be exposed with high probability for five or more years. Phthalates are immunologically active, inducing allergic responses such as "meat wrapper's asthma" in susceptible individuals. Workers exposed to phthalic anhydrides have elevated levels of IgE and/or IgG specific to that phthalate (Topping 1986; Nielsen 1988; Flaherty 1988). Plastic implants have also induced plasmacytoma in rodents. These data suggest that studies in occupational populations with likely exposure to immunologically active substances may provide additional leads to myeloma etiology.

In summary, results of this population-based case-control study of myeloma among Danish men suggest increases in risk of myeloma with exposure to gasoline or engine exhausts and to phthalate plasticizers. Given the large number of industries and occupations evaluated, these could be chance findings. Associations were not strong, but are consistent with some previous studies. The findings should be interpreted cautiously, but suggest avenues that could be explored fruitfully by other researchers.

REFERENCES

Cuzick J, De Stavola B (1988) Multiple myeloma - a case-control study. Br J Cancer 57:516-520

Delzell E, Monson RR (1985) Mortality among rubber workers: X. Reclaim workers. Am J Indus Med 7:307-313

Flaherty DK, Gross CJ, Winzenburger P, Comps MB, McGarity K, Tillman E (1988) In vitro immunologic studies on a population of workers exposed to phthalic and tetrachlorophthalic anhydride. J Occup Med 30:785-790

Flodin U, Fredriksson M, Persson B (1987) Multiple myeloma and engine exhausts, fresh wood, and creosote: a case referent study. Am J Indus Med 12:519-529

Greene MH, Hoover RN, Eck RL, et al (1979) Cancer mortality among printing plant workers. Environ Res 20:66-74

Lundberg I (1986) Mortality and cancer incidence among Swedish paint industry workers with long-term exposure to organic solvents. Scand J Work Environ Health 12:108-113

Monson RR, Nakano KK (1976) Mortality among rubber workers. II. Other employees. Am J Epidemiol 103:297

Morris PD, Koepsell TD, Daling JR, et al (1986) Toxic substance exposure and multiple myeloma: a case-control study. J Natl Cancer Inst 76:987-994

Nielsen J, Welinder H, Schutz A, Skerfving S (1988) Specific serum antibodies against phthalic anhydride in occupationally exposed subjects. J Allergy Clin Immunol 82:126-133

Riedel DA, Pottern LM, Blattner WA (1990) The epidemiology of multiple myeloma. In: Wiernik PH, Canellos GP, Kyle RA, Schiffer CA (eds) Neoplastic diseases of the blood, 2nd edn. Churchill Livingstone, New York, in press

Topping MD, Venables KM, Luczynska CM, Howe W, Newman Taylor AJ (1986) Specificity of the human IgE response to inhaled acid anhydrides. J Allergy Clin Immunol 77:834-842

Familial and Genetic Associations

A.F. Olshan

Department of Clinical Epidemiology and Preventive Medicine,
University of Pittsburgh, M200 Scaife Hall,
Pittsburgh, PA 15261

INTRODUCTION

Research with animals has indicated that there is a genetic component in the etiology of multiple myeloma (this volume). Human studies have also provided some clues to the genetic basis of the disease. Given the paucity of known environmental risk factors for multiple myeloma an understanding of the role that genetic factors may play is crucial. Genetic factors may help explain the increased incidence of multiple myeloma in blacks as compared with whites.

The purpose of this report is to review the epidemiologic characteristics of familial multiple myeloma, the familial aggregation of cancer and other diseases, and the association with genetic markers. Directions for future research will also be suggested.

RESULTS

Familial Multiple Myeloma

The data on familial multiple myeloma was obtained from the excellent review by Blattner (1980) and the published reports listed in Table 1. The published reports of familial multiple myeloma (1954-1987) include a total of 104 cases in 49 families. The majority of families included sibs (66%) and parent-offspring (25%) cases. Other familial relationships were cousins (4%), aunt-niece (2%), and uncle-nephew (3%) sets. A study at the Mayo Clinic reported 8 familial cases among a total of 440 multiple myeloma cases diagnosed in 6 years (Maldanado and Kyle, 1974). Only one black familial case of multiple myeloma has been reported. The mode of inheritance is thought to be autosomal recessive (McKusick, 1988) although poor ascertainment in previous generations could mask other modes of transmission.

The sex distribution for familial cases (56% male) was similar to sporadic cases (51% male). Figure 1 shows the age distribution of familial cases compared with the data from the Surveillance, End Results, and Epidemiology (SEER) program (National Cancer Institute, 1989). The familial cases had a younger age at diagnosis than the SEER cases. The median age at diagnosis for familial cases was 63 years compared to 70 years for SEER cases. A similar age pattern was found for males and females. However, the median age at diagnosis for cases seen at the Mayo Clinic is 62 years (R. Kyle, personal communication). The average age at diagnosis differed by 21 years for parent-offspring sets and 9 years for sibs. The average number of years between diagnoses was 21 years for parent-offspring cases and 6 years among sibs.

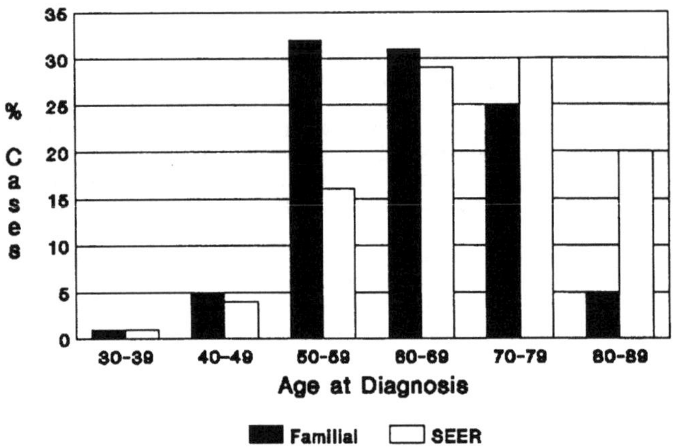

Fig. 1. Distribution of age at diagnosis for familial cases compared with cases from the SEER program

Figure 2 presents the distribution of immunoglobulin classes for familial cases and 710 cases diagnosed at the Mayo Clinic 1982-1988 (R. Kyle, personal communication). The class distributions were similar expect for a slight excess of IgA among familial cases. The kappa/lambda ratios for familial cases compared with the Mayo Clinic data is shown in Figure 3. The ratios are slightly higher for familial cases among all classes. Fourteen of the families included cases of concurrent multiple myeloma. The concordance of heavy chain class among familial cases was 47% (9/19) and 79% (11/14) concordance for light chain type. Blattner (1980) has suggested that the concordance of light-chain type was genetically-based, while an elevated kappa-lambda ratio may indicate an altered antibody pattern in familial cases.

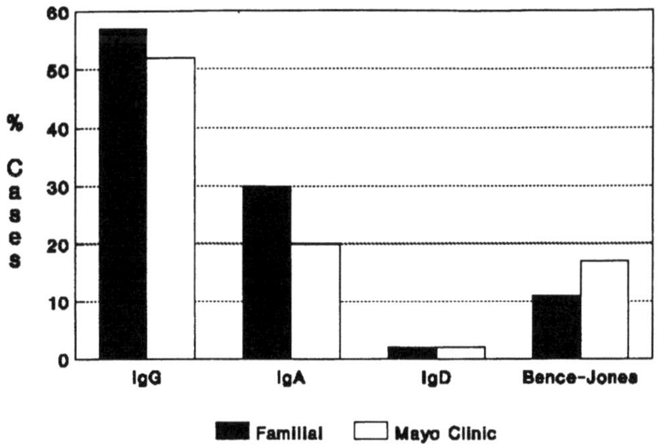

Fig. 2. Distribution of immunoglobulin classes for familial cases and cases from the Mayo Clinic

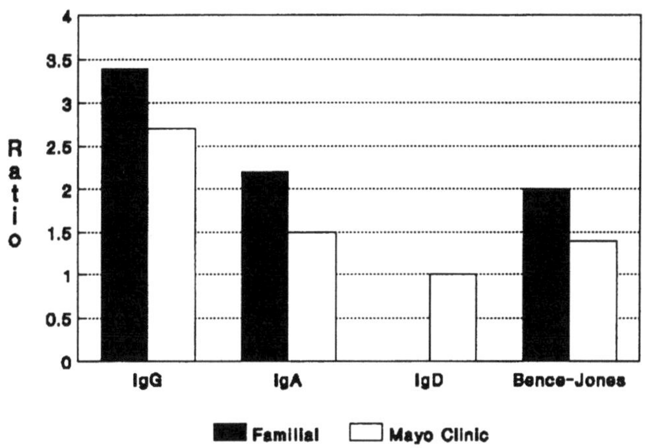

Fig. 3. Kappa/lambda ratios for immunoglobulin classes. Familial cases compared with Mayo Clinic cases.

There have been three twin pairs concordant for multiple myeloma reported in the literature. The first monozygotic twin pair was diagnosed in England (Judson et al, 1985). The diagnoses were made within two years of each other and both twins had IgG kappa myeloma. Both brothers had lived and worked together unloading ships at London docks. In second monozygotic twin pair, one twin's disease was IgA lambda, while the other twin had free kappa light chain (McCrea et al, 1986). The third pair, possibly monozygotic, were diagnosed 8 years apart, one with free kappa light-chain and the other with kappa IgG (Comotti et al, 1987). The twins had lived and worked separately since age 21 years.

An interesting immunogenetic study of two brothers with multiple myeloma and their relatives was recently reported (Grosbois et al., 1986). The brothers were diagnosed 6 months apart and both were IgG kappa. The brothers shared identical HLA genotypes (A2 B12 DR4/A9 B27 DR2). There was no HLA genotype identity with the brothers among 34 other family members tested. Nine family members were semi-identical for haplotype a and 5 for haplotype d. There were no other cases of monoclonal gammopathy in the family members examined.

Familial Aggregation of Disease

There have been several reports of an excess of various diseases in the relatives of patients with multiple myeloma. Familial aggregation of cancer, autoimmune disorders and degenerative CNS diseases has been found. A case-control study of 439 cases and 1317 hospital controls at Duke University found an association with cancer in any first-degree relative (odds ratio (OR)=1.4; 95% confidence interval (CI)= 1.1-1.8) (Bourguet et al., 1985). If the age at diagnosis of multiple myeloma was less than 50 years of age, the association with any cancer among first-degree relatives was stronger (OR=2.5; CI=1.1 -5.3). The relative risk associated with a first-degree relative with cancer of the lymphatic and hematopoietic system was 2.4 (CI=1.4- 4.0). Associations were also found for a family history of gastrointestinal cancer (OR=1.3; CI=0.9- 1.8, lung cancer (OR=1.7; CI=1.0- 2.9), breast cancer (OR=1.3; CI=0.8- 2.1), and genitourinary cancer (OR=1.5; CI=0.9-2.4). There were insufficient data available to analyze family history separately among black cases. A case-control study of 100 cases and 100 hospital controls in Baltimore (Linet et al., 1988) found an excess among first-degree relatives of leukemia (OR=3.0), breast cancer (OR=2.7), endometrial cancer (4 cases/0 controls), cancer of the buccal cavity and pharynx (OR=2.0), stomach cancer (OR=1.7), and lung cancer (OR=1.7).

The Baltimore case-control study also found an association with a prior history of rheumatoid arthritis and subsequent development of multiple myeloma. This finding is consistent with some previous studies (Isomaki et al., 1978; Katusic et al, 1985; Hakulinen et al, 1985; Pearce et al, 1986), but not all others (Cohen et al, 1987; Cuzick and De Stavola, 1988). Linet et al (1988) further evaluated the association with rheumatoid arthritis by examining the history of autoimmune disorders among first-degree relatives. An association with family history of any autoimmune disorder was observed (OR=3.0; CI=1.3- 7.1). The association was explained by an excess of rheumatoid arthritis among relatives (OR=3.7; CI=1.0- 13.1). Weaker associations were also detected for family history of systemic lupus erythematosus and pernicious anemia.

The possible relationship between multiple myeloma and family history of central nervous system diseases was examined using data from the Duke University case-control study described above (Grufferman et al, 1989). The hypothesis for this analysis came from an earlier observation that relatives of patients with early-onset Alzheimer's disease had an increased risk of Down syndrome and myeloproliferative disorders, including multiple myeloma (Heston, 1977). Thirteen of the 439 cases and 9 of 1317 controls had one or more first-degree relatives with a degenerative or demyelinating central nervous system disease (OR=4.4; CI=1.9- 10.3). Analysis by specific disease category resulted in increased relative risks for Parkinson's disease (OR=3.0; CI=0.9- 10.3), multiple sclerosis (OR=4.0; CI=0.9-17.8) and a small residual category that included other degenerative or demyelinating CNS diagnoses (OR=11.9; CI=1.3-107.1). Only one familial occurrence of Alzheimer's disease was found.

Association with Genetic Markers

A review of the literature on HLA antigens and multiple myeloma found that 4 studies reported an association with HLA-B5, with relative risks ranging from 2 to 66 (Miller, 1974; Mason and Cullen, 1975; Festen et al, 1976; Cassuto et al, 1981). Elevated, but non-statistically significant relative risks for HLA-B5 were reported in two studies (Smith et al, 1974; Jeannet et al, 1976). Five studies did not find any association with the HLA-B5 antigen (Bertrams et al, 1972; Van Camp et al, 1977; Saleun et al, 1979; Tannov, 1981; Ludwig and Mayr, 1982). Two studies (Bertrams et al, 1972; Smith et al, 1974) detected an association with the B18 antigen. Ludwig and Mayr (1982) performed a combined analysis of pooled data from the literature (379 cases and 5041 controls). The only association found was with the B5 antigen (weighted relative risk= 1.7). A similar combined analysis of HLA-B5 found an increase, but also some heterogeneity in the pooled data (Tiwari and Terasaki, 1985). There are little data available on the population association of the D loci and multiple myeloma. One study (Muylle, 1982) of 28 patients found no association with HLA-DR antigens.

In one of the few genetic studies of multiple myeloma among blacks a strong association was found with the HLA-Cw5 antigen (4 of 22 cases/2 of 138 controls; OR=15) (Leech et al, 1983). A weaker relationship was obtained for the Cw6 antigen (OR= 6.5). All four multiple myeloma cases with the Cw5 antigen were males.

The immunoglobulin allotypes, Gm and Km, have also been examined for their possible association with multiple myeloma. The Gm and Km allotypes are polymorphic markers for the constant regions of the heavy chain of subclasses of IgG, IgA, IgE and the kappa light chains, respectively. An Austrian study of 68 cases (Ludwig and Mayr, 1982) found an association with the G1m(x) allotype (OR=2.1).

Their combined analysis of allotype data from the literature [258 cases/ 4550 controls; allotypes G1m a, x, f, Km(1)] did not detect an association with any allotype, including G1m(x). Leech et al (1985) examined the Gm allotype series in their sample of 29 black multiple myeloma cases and 160 black control subjects and found a strong association with G3m(g5) (93% of cases, 47% of controls; OR=15). The authors conclude that the G3m(g5) allotype is a marker of inherited susceptibility to multiple myeloma among blacks. The specific mechanism or role of the allotype in the pathogenesis of multiple myeloma is not known.

Directions for Future Research

There are several leads that have been generated from the study of familial aggregation of disease and association with genetic markers. The families of patients with multiple myeloma are at increased risk of a variety of conditions including cancer, autoimmune disease, and degenerative CNS diseases. These findings from two studies clearly need to be replicated. New studies should include a larger sample, careful attention should be paid to the choice of comparison groups, and validation of reported familial disease undertaken. In addition, new techniques for the analysis of familial aggregation of disease using case-control data should be incorporated (Liang, 1987). Where possible, immunogenetic and other marker data should be obtained from family members. The study of the population association of HLA and allotype markers with multiple myeloma has produced a few positive results. Many of these early studies had very small samples and did not include all antigens now available (eg., HLA-D loci). New developments with restriction fragment polymorphisms may open up new areas of study (Ghanem et al, 1989) for population and family studies.

Given the increased incidence of multiple myeloma among blacks, the need for further study in this group is apparent. Studies of familial aggregation of disease in blacks have not been attempted. The studies of genetic markers among blacks by Leech and colleagues have provided some interesting and potentially important findings that warrant further examination.

Table 1. Familial multiple myeloma cases reported after 1980.

Year	Reference	Relationship	Age	Immunoglobulin Type[a]	
1982	Shoenfeld	Mother	78	IgG λ	
		Son	63	IgG λ	
1985	Horwitz	Sister	53	BJ κ	
		Sister	51	IgG κ	
		Sister	56	IgG κ	
1985	Bourget	Brother	75	IgA λ	
		Brother	50		
		Brother	47	IgA κ	
		Sister	53		
		Sister	70	IgG λ	
		Sister			
1985	Judson	Brother	61	IgG κ	Twin
		Brother	63	IgG κ	Twin
1986	Grosbois	Brother	61	IgG κ	
		Brother	63	IgG κ	
1986	Rostoker	Mother	84	IgG κ	
		Daughter	60	IgG κ	
1986	McCrea	Father	82	IgG κ	
		Son	53	IgG	
		Mother	83	IgA κ	
		Daughter	52	BJ κ	
		Brother	58	IgA κ	Twin
		Brother	61	BJ κ	Twin
1987	Comotti	Sister	60	BJ κ	Twin
		Sister	68	IgG κ	Twin

[a] BJ= Bence Jones light chain

REFERENCES

Bertrams J, Kuwert E, Böhme U, Reis HE, Gallmeier WM, Wetter O, Schmidt CG (1972) HL-A antigens in Hodgkin's disease and multiple myeloma. Tissue Antigens 2:41-46

Blattner WA (1980) Multiple myeloma and related plasma cell disorders: an analytic review. Progress in Myeloma 1-65

Bourguet CC, Grufferman S, Delzell E, Delong ER, Cohen HJ (1985) Multiple myeloma and family history of cancer. Cancer 56:2133-2139

Cassuto JP, Piereschi J, Maiolini R, Dujardin O, Ribeil R, Masseyeff R (1981) Marqueurs HLA dans les myelomes et les dysglobulinemies monoclonales benignes. Nouv Presse Med 10:252-253

Cohen HJ, Bernstein RJ, Grufferman (1987) Role of immune stimulation in the etiology of multiple myeloma: A case control study. Am J Hemat 24:119-126

Comotti B, Bassan R, Buzzetti M, Finazzi G, Barbui T (1987) Multiple myeloma in a pair of twins. British Journal of Haematology 65:123-124

Festen JJM, Marrink J, Sijpesteijn JAK, Loghem EV, Nijenhuis LE, Mandema E (1976) A study on the association between myelomatosis and immunoglobulin allotypes, HLA, and blood groups. Immunogenetics 3:201-203

Ghanem N, Dugoujon JM, Lefranc MP, Lefranc G (1989) BstEII restriction fragment alleles and haplotypes of the human IGHG genes with reference to the BamHI/SacI RFLPs and to the gm polymorphism. Expl Clin Immunogenet 6:39-54

Grosbois B, Gueguen M, Fauchet R, Lebouc H, Guenot A, Lancelin F, Lauvin R, Lebouc H, Leblay R, Genetet B (1986) Multiple myeloma in two brothers. Cancer 58:2417-2421

Grufferman S, Cohen HJ, Delzell ES, Morrison MC, Schold SC Jr., Moore JO (1989) Familial aggregation of multiple myeloma and central nervous system diseases. J Am Geriatr Soc 37:303-309

Hakulinen T, Isomaki H, Knekt P (1985) Rheumatoid arthritis and cancer studies. Am J Med 78(1A):29-32

Heston LL, Mastri Ar, Anderson VE (1981) Dementia of the Alzheimer type: clinical genetics, natural history and associated conditions. Arch Gen Psychiatry 38:1085-1090

Horwitz LJ, Levy RN, Rosner F (1985) Multiple myeloma in three siblings. Arch Intern Med 145:1449-1450

Isomaki HA, Hakulinen T, Joutsenlahti U (1978) Excess risk of lymphomas, leukemia and myeloma in patients with rheumatoid arthritis. J Chron Dis 31:691-696

Jeannet M, Magnin C (1976) HL-A antigen in haematological malignant disease. Eur J Clin Invest 2:39-42

Judson IR, Wiltshaw E, Newland AC (1985) Multiple myeloma in a pair of monozygotic twins: the first reported case. British Journal of Haematology 60:551-554

Katusic S, Beard CM, Kurland LT, Weis JW, Bergstrahl E (1985) Occurrence of malignant neoplasms in the Rochester, Minnesota, rheumatoid arthritis cohort. Am J Med 78(1A):50-55

Leech SH, Brown R, Schanfield MS (1985) Genetic studies in multiple myeloma. II. Immunoglobulin allotype associations. Cancer 55:1473-1476

Leech SH, Bryan CF, Elston RC, Rainey J, Bickers JN, Pelias MZ (1983) Genetic studies in multiple myeloma. Association with HLA cw5. Cancer 51:1408-1411

Liang Ky (1987) Extended Mantel-Haenszel estimating procedure for multivariate logistic regression models. Biometrics 43:289-299
Linet MS, McLaughlin JK, Harlow SD, Fraumeni JF (1988) Family history of autoimmune disorders and cancer in multiple myeloma. Int J Epidemiol 17:512-513
Ludwig H, Mayr W (1982) Genetic aspects of susceptibility to multiple myeloma. Blood 59:1286-1291
Maldonado JE, Kyle RA (1974) Familial myeloma. Am J Med 57:875-884
Mason DY, Cullen P (1975) HL-A antigen frequencies in myeloma. Tissue Antigens 5:238-245
McCrea AP, Morris TCM (1986) Concurrent familial myeloma in Northern Ireland. Cancer 58:394-396
McKusick VA (1988) Mendelian inheritance in man: Catologs of autosomal dominant, autosomal recessive and X-linked phenotypes, ed. 5. Baltimore: The Johns Hopkins University Press 1088-1089
Miller WV (1974) HL-A antigens and hematologic malignancy. Arch Intern Med 133:397-399
Muylle L, DeSmet D, Cole J, Peetermans ME (1982) HLA-DR and monoclonal gammapathy. Tissue Antigens 20:397-399
Pearce NE, Smith AH, Howard JK, Sheppard RA, Giles HJ, Teague CA (1986) Case-control study of multiple myeloma and farming. Br J Cancer 54:493-500
Rostoker G, Uzzan B, Baumelou E, Chapman A (1986) Myélome familial IgG kappa chez une mére et sa fille. Nouv Rev Fr Hematol 28:27-32
Saleün JP, Youinou P, LeGoff P, LeMenn G, Morin JF (1979) HLA antigens and monoclonal gammapathy. Tissue Antigens 13:233-235
Shoenfeld Y, Shaklai M, Berliner S, Gallant LA, Pinkhas J (1982) Familial multiple myeloma. A review of thirty-seven families. Postgrad Med J 58:12-16
Smith G, Walford RL, Fishkin B, Carter PK, Tanaka K (1974) HL-A phenotypes, immunoglobulins and K and L chains in multiple myeloma. Tissue Antigens 4:374-377
Tananov AT, Kutyina RM, Turbina NS, Abakumov EM, Polyanskaya Am, Isaev VG (1981) HLA antigens in patients with blood pathology. Prob Gematol Pereliv Krovi 26:8-12
Tiwari L, Terasaki PI (1985) HLA and disease associations. Springer-Verlag, New York
Van Camp BGK, Cole J, Peetermans ME (1977) HLA antigens and homogeneous immunoglobulins. Clinical Immunology and Immunopathology 7:315-318

Black/White Differences in Risk

Racial Variations in Immune Function and Hematological Parameters: Description of Study Design and Objectives

L.M. Brown, D.J. Tollerud*, W.A. Blattner, and R.N. Hoover

National Cancer Institute, Epidemiology and Biostatistics Program, Executive Plaza North Room 415, Bethesda, MD 20892.

* Department of Occupational and Environmental Health, Graduate School of Public Health, University of Pittsburgh, Pittsburgh, PA.

INTRODUCTION

This paper describes a population-based study conducted by the National Cancer Institute which included the collection of blood from healthy black and white adults in the Washington, DC area and their children. For logistical reasons the initial survey excluded interviews with black smokers.

Data from this survey was used to describe immunologic and hematologic differences between black and white nonsmokers possibly related to the black excess of multiple myeloma. Presented in this paper is a general overview of study concerns, objectives, and design.

There are significant methodologic concerns encountered in conducting a population-based study with a biochemical component. These include: 1) population selection and recruitment, 2) confidentiality and quality control of the information collected, and 3) logistics of blood collection and handling. Investigators must weigh the advantages of using a population-based sample against the difficulties involved in collecting biologic specimens from a representative sample of the general population.

Our study conducted from May 1984 through September 1984 was designed to investigate the influence of demographic, lifestyle and medical factors on T-cell subsets. Since previous reports of "normal" T-cell values came from small or highly selected populations such as laboratory volunteers, or blood donors, we decided to collect blood and questionnaire information from a population-based sample of healthy adults in order to obtain a clearer understanding of the range of "normal" values in the general population.

Our goal was to obtain valid questionnaire and blood data for ten healthy adults in each of 30 age-sex-race-smoking strata. To obtain a representative study sample, our study design utilized three phases. Phase I - selection of households and potential study subjects by random digit dialing (RDD); Phase II - telephone interviews and selection of study subjects medically eligible for blood collection; and Phase III - self-administered interviews, blood collection, and selection of final study sample.

PHASE I -

In Phase I, random digit dialing (RDD) was used to select a random sample of households based on telephone exchanges which approximated the

Maryland-Washington, DC-Virginia Standard Metropolitan Statistical Area (SMSA). A 5 minute household screening questionnaire was used to obtain the name, sex, age, race, and smoking status of all household members and to ascertain eligible adults aged 20-69. A total of 3888 households completed this short questionnaire for a response rate of 83%. Using sampling fractions established by race-sex-age-and smoking status, 1043 household members were selected to participate in Phase II of the study.

PHASE II

Phase II involved administration of a 25 minute telephone questionnaire which was designed to collect basic demographic, occupational, smoking, beverage, and medical information. It was also used to exclude subjects with medical conditions which might alter T-cell subsets from further participation in the study. A total of 849 subjects completed the telephone questionnaire for a response rate of 81%. The race-sex specific response rates were 83% for white males, 88% for white females, 72% for black males and 74% for black females. Two hundred forty six subjects (29%) were medically ineligible for participation in Phase III of the study because they met at least one of the following medical exclusionary criteria. They had been treated for severe allergies or hospitalized during the past 3 months; had taken steroid medication during the past year; had received a blood transfusion since 1975; had been told by a doctor that they had SLE, rheumatoid arthritis, a severe bleeding disorder, or cancer; or were recently or currently pregnant.

PHASE III

The 603 subjects determined to be medically eligible for Phase III were sent a letter inviting them to complete a short questionnaire and have a blood specimen taken at a mobile van parked at a hospital in their area. Participating adults with children between the ages of 12 and 19 were asked to bring one or two children to answer a short health questionnaire and have a blood sample taken. Each participating family member would be paid $25.00 for giving blood and each family would receive $10.00 for transportation. Remuneration of study subjects for the inconvenience involved was considered necessary to attract healthy subjects to enroll in this phase of the study. Use of a mobile van parked at 11 different locations minimized the burden on respondents, while providing a centrally located facility for interviews, blood collection, and blood processing.

In the van, subjects had their blood drawn by a registered nurse for routine clinical laboratory tests and for analysis of T-cell subsets. Each of the three types of blood specimens collected: anticoagulated blood, heparinized blood, and serum required its own protocol for handling and processing. Adults also completed a 15 minute two-part self-administered questionnaire. The first part of the questionnaire obtained recent smoking, alcohol, dietary, and medical histories. The second part collected personal lifestyle information concerning illicit drug use and homosexual activity. The information from these questionnaires was used to further exclude subjects with conditions which might affect the immunolgic parameters under investigation. The number of participating adults was 401 or 67%. White males gave blood most often (75%), followed by white females (72%), black males (57%) and black females (45%). After excluding subjects for medical reasons or laboratory error, the final study population consisted of 374 adult subjects and 112 children.

The Influence of Race on T-Cell Subset Distributions

David J. Tollerud[1], Linda Morris Brown, William A. Blattner, and Robert N. Hoover

Epidemiology and Biometry Program, National Cancer Institute, Bethesda, MD.

SUMMARY

To investigate the influence of race on the cellular immune system, we analyzed peripheral blood mononuclear cell subsets in 266 healthy nonsmoking adults and 112 healthy children. Among adults, blacks had a significantly higher proportion of B cells, a lower proportion of T cells, and a higher proportion of HLA-DR positive cells and activated T cells than whites. Among children, the proportion of HLA-DR positive cells and activated T cells were significantly higher in blacks than in whites, but the proportion of T cells and B cells were similar in blacks and whites. An apparent decrease in the proportion of CD4+ (T-Helper) cells was observed in black women age 50 and older compared to white women and younger black women. These and other race-related immunologic alterations may provide clues to the etiology of diseases and conditions which exhibit significant racial differences.

INTRODUCTION

Recent investigations have demonstrated that the immune system is quantitatively and qualitatively affected by numerous host factors, medical conditions and environmental exposures. Age, gender, allergies and exposure to cigarette smoke, for example, have all been associated with distinct alterations in T-cell subset distributions. Much less is known about the influence of race or ethnic background on the immune system. Blacks are known to have a lower leukocyte count due a relative decrease in neutrophils compared to whites (Karayalcian, Rosner and Sawitsky 1972; Van Assendelft 1985). Blacks are also reported to have a higher average IgE level than whites (Grundbacher 1975). Prince and colleagues reported significant race-related differences in T-cell subsets and natural killer cells between Asians and whites but found no significant differences for the limited number of blacks in the study (Prince, Hirji, Waldbeser et al. 1985). To address potential black:white differences in the cellular immune system, we analyzed peripheral blood mononuclear cell subsets in a population-based sample of healthy adults and their children (Tollerud, Clark, Brown et al. 1989; Tollerud, Ildstad, Brown 1990).

---

1 Current Address: University of Pittsburgh Graduate School of Public Health Room A-718, Pittsburgh, PA 15261

METHODS

The study population was selected by random digit dialing from households in the Washington, D.C. metropolitan area. After screening to determine demographic characteristics and cigarette smoking status, a detailed questionnaire was administered to exclude individuals with illnesses, exposures or medical conditions which might affect the immunological parameters under investigation. The analyses presented here were limited to black and white nonsmoking adults and a sample of children ages 12-19 from the study households.

The following directly fluorescein conjugated monoclonal antibodies, purchased from Ortho Diagnostics, Raritan, NJ (ORTHO) or Becton Dickinson Monoclonal Center, Mountain View, CA (BD) were used in the analyses: OKT3 (CD3+ T-cells; ORTHO); OKT4 and OKT4A (CD4+ helper-inducer T-cell subset; ORTHO); OKT8 (CD8+ suppressor-cytotoxic T-cell subset; ORTHO); anti-Leu 12 (CD19+ B-cells; BD); anti-Leu M3 (CD14+ monocytes; BD); anti-Leu 11A (CD16+ natural killer cells; BD); anti HLA-DR (nonpolymorphic HLA-DR antigen; BD); and mouse IgG1 (clone 11-63; BD) and IgG(a+b) (clones 11-4.1 and MPC-11; BD) as negative control reagents. Single parameter flow cytometry analyses were performed on a FACS II cell sorter (BD, Mountain View, CA) using forward and right-angle light scatter gating. The relative proportion of activated T-cells (ACT-T) was estimated by subtracting from the HLA-DR+ cell pool the number of B-cells and the number of monocytes not eliminated by right-angle-scatter gating. Linear regression analysis was employed to evaluate the relative contributions of age, race, gender, and other independent variables on mononuclear cell subset proportions.

RESULTS AND DISCUSSION

The black:white differences we observed are summarized in Table 1. Among adults, blacks had a higher proportion of B cells, a lower proportion of T cells, and a higher proportion of HLA-DR+ cells than whites. The estimated proportion of activated T cells was also significantly higher in blacks than in whites and increased significantly with age (Fig. 1). Among the children, the increase in CD3+ cells among whites was not statistically significant, and there was no significant difference in CD19+ cells (Table 1). Like adults, black children had significantly higher levels of HLA-DR+ cells and activated T cells. Further analysis of gender and age strata also revealed that black women age 50 or older had a significantly lower proportion of CD4+ (T-Helper) cells compared to white women and younger black women ($p<0.05$) (Fig. 2). No such discontinuity was observed for men. No significant differences in CD8+ (T-Suppressor/Cytotoxic) cells, CD16+ (Natural Killer) cells or CD14+ cells (monocytes) between blacks and whites.

One additional black:white difference confirmed in these studies was the previously reported heterogeneity of the T4 epitope of the CD4 cell surface antigen among blacks (Fuller, Trevithick, Fuller et al. 1984) (Fig. 3). The inheritance pattern has been shown to be a Mendelian co-dominant pattern, with a similar distribution of phenotypes among black populations world-wide. Affected individuals have normal numbers of CD4+ cells, and no functional differences associated with the T4 epitope heterogeneity have been reported.

Table 1. Black:White Differences in Mononuclear Cell Subsets[1]

Cell Surface Antigen	Whites	Blacks	p Value[2]
ADULTS			
CD3 (T cells)	76.1 ± 0.05	73.6 ± 0.8	< 0.01
CD19 (B cells)	10.0 ± 0.3	11.8 ± 0.4	< 0.001
HLA-DR	14.0 ± 0.4	17.9 ± 0.6	≤ 0.0001
"ACT-T"[3]	2.1 ± 0.4	4.0 ± 0.6	≤ 0.0001
CHILDREN			
CD3 (T cells)	74.7 ± 0.7	72.1 ± 1.5	NS
CD19 (B cells)	10.1 ± 0.6	9.4 ± 1.0	NS
HLA-DR	14.8 ± 0.5	17.1 ± 1.1	< 0.05
"ACT-T"[3]	2.8 ± 0.6	6.0 ± 1.0	≤ 0.01

[1]Values expressed as mean ± SE percentage of lymphoid cells
[2]p value from multiple linear regression model adjusting for the influence of age and gender. NS: $p > 0.05$
[3]ACT-T is a derived estimate of the proportion of circulating activated T-cells

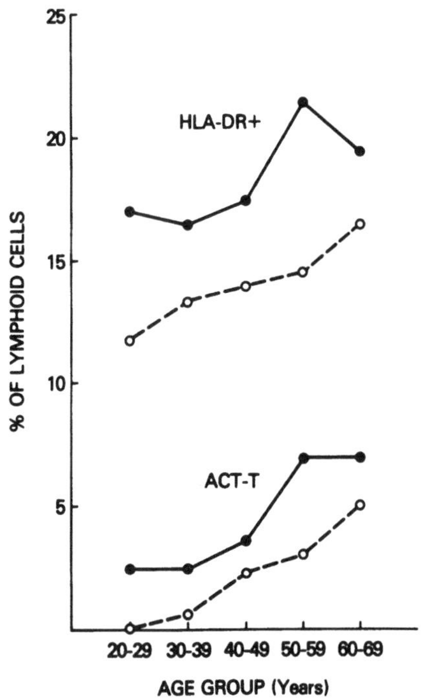

Figure 1: Influence of race and age on HLA-DR+ cells and activated T cells (ACT-T). Solid circles = black subjects; open circles = white subjects. $p \leq 0.0001$ for blacks versus whites. (From Tollerud, Clark, Brown et al. 1989)

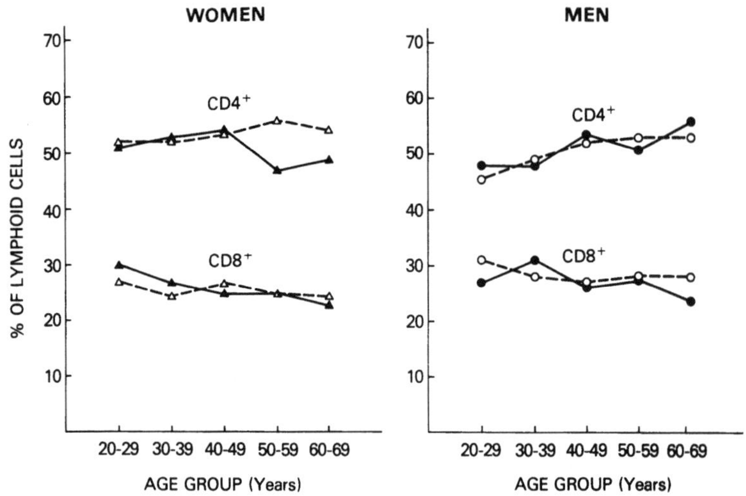

Figure 2: Influence of race and age on T-cell subsets in men and women. Solid triangles = black women; open triangles = white women; solid circles = black men; open circles = white men. (Adapted from Tollerud, Clark, Brown et al. 1989)

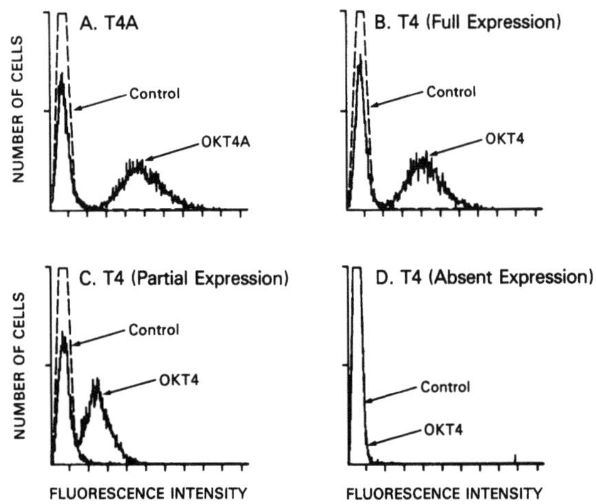

Figure 3: Differential expression of the T4 epitope in blacks and whites. A. Typical fluorescence intensity histogram for cells labeled with OKT4A; B. Full expression of the T4 epitope (100% of whites, 50-70% of blacks); Partial Expression (22-39% of blacks); and Absent Expression (4-11% of blacks). (From Tollerud et al. 1989 and 1990)

The clinical significance of these race-related differences remains uncertain. To date, no significant functional differences in immunologic responses have been reported for different racial groups. Even the dramatically lower neutrophil count among blacks compared to whites has no known clinical correlates. However, these data emphasize that there are clear-cut differences between blacks and whites for a variety of immunologic parameters. Present data do not permit a clear distinction between genetic and environmental effects underlying these differences. Future efforts should be directed at determining whether such immunologic differences may play a role in those diseases and conditions which show distinct racial differences in incidence or severity.

REFERENCES

Fuller TC, Trevithick JE, Fuller AA, Colvin RB, Cosimi AB, Kung PC (1984) Antigenic polymorphism of the T4 differentiation antigen expressed on human T helper/inducer lymphocytes. Human Immunol 9: 89-102.

Grundbacher FJ (1975) Causes of variation in serum IgE levels in normal populations. J All Clin Immunol 56: 104-111.

Karayalcian G, Rosner F, Sawitsky A (1972) Pseudoneutropenia in Negroes: A normal phenomenon. N Y State J Med 72: 1815-1817.

Prince HE, Hirji K, Waldbeser LS, Plaeger-Marshall S, Klinman S, Lanier LL (1985) Influence of racial background with distribution of T-cell subsets and Leu 11-positive lymphocytes in healthy blood donors. Diagn Immunol 3: 33-37.

Tollerud DJ, Clark JW, Brown LM, Neuland CY, Pankiw-Trost LK, Blattner WA, Hoover RN (1989) The influence of age, race, and gender on peripheral blood mononuclear cell subsets in healthy nonsmokers. J Clin Immunol 9: 214-222.

Tollerud DJ, Ildstad ST, Brown LM, Clark JW, Blattner WA, Mann DL, Neuland CY, Pankiw-Trost L, Hoover RN (1990) T-cell subsets in healthy teenagers: transition to the adult phenotype. Clin Immunol Immunopathol 1990 (In Press).

Van Assendelft OW (1985) Reference values for the total and differential leukocyte count. Blood Cells 11: 77-96.

Investigating Risk Factors for Multiple Myeloma among Black and White Americans

L.M. Pottern

Environmental Epidemiology Branch;, National Cancer Institute, NIH, Executive Plaza North, Suite 418, Bethesda, MD 20892

INTRODUCTION

Racial variations in the incidence of various cancer types can provide important etiologic leads for epidemiologists to pursue. The fact that multiple myeloma is the only hematopoietic malignancy which occurs more frequently among U.S. blacks than whites has been especially intriguing to researchers at the National Cancer Institute. To investigate reasons for the black-white differences in risk for multiple myeloma (and three other cancer types), a large-scale epidemiologic study was initiated in 1985. This study was a collaborative endeavor involving the National Cancer Institute, the Georgia Center for Cancer Statistics, the Michigan Cancer Foundation, and the New Jersey State Health Department.

This paper provides a brief overview of the study design and risk factors under investigation. There were several unique design aspects of our study. This study is the first population-based case-control study designed to identify race-specific risk factors for four cancer types which have higher rates among blacks than whites. Using a special rapid-reporting system, cases of multiple myeloma and the other cancers were identified among both black and white Americans from over 150 hospitals in the three study areas. A modular questionnaire was developed so that subjects with each of the four cancer types could be asked a specific set of questions while the control group could be asked all of the questions. In this way, one control group rather than four can be used in the risk analysis of each cancer type. Another unique aspect of the study is the inclusion of a biochemical component. For the male multiple myeloma cases and controls, differences in human leukocyte antigens (HLA) between blacks and whites will be examined as potential markers of genetic susceptibility.

METHODS

Selection of Study Population

The study population included all cases of multiple myeloma among blacks and whites, aged 30-79, newly diagnosed over the time period 1986-1989 from three areas of the U.S.: Atlanta, Detroit and New Jersey. Controls were frequency-matched to the cases on five-year age categories within race/gender groups. The number of population controls to be sampled was determined based on the age-race-sex distribution of previously diagnosed cases from each study area. Random digit dialing (RDD) techniques were used in selecting controls less than 65 years of age. Controls aged 65 years and older were selected from the Health Care Finance Administrations' computerized tapes of medicare recipients.

Study Procedures

Hospitals in each of the three study areas were visited on a periodic basis to identify cases from records in the pathology and hematology department and out-patient clinics. Our goal was to interview cases within three months of diagnosis. Once a case was identified, the patient's physician was contacted to obtain permission to interview the case and draw blood.

An introductory letter was sent to all subjects which was followed by a phone call to schedule an interview. Interviews were conducted with the subject at home by a trained interviewer. At the end of the interview, all male cases and selected male controls were asked to participate in the blood component of the study. A phlebotomist called the subject to answer any questions and arrange for the blood drawing at the subject's home. Prior to blood drawing, the phlebotomist obtained signed consent and administered a short questionnaire. After taking the blood specimen, the phlebotomist promptly returned to the lab to process the blood samples. The white cells were then shipped in transport media within 24 hours to a laboratory in Washington, D.C., where the HLA typing was conducted.

Potential Risk Factors

Our questionnaire was designed to ascertain information on all suspected and potential risk factors for multiple myeloma. It included questions on sociodemographic characteristics to clarify conflicting evidence to date of an association between socioeconomic status and multiple myeloma.

Detailed questions on lifestyle factors such as tobacco use, alcoholic beverage consumption, and usual adult dietary history, were asked in the questionnaire. These factors have not been previously explored in depth and could differentially contribute to myeloma risk by race. The questionnaire also contained an extensive medical history section which focused on infectious, autoimmune and chronic diseases and allergies in an attempt to confirm an apriori hypothesis that chronic antigenic stimulation plays a role in the development of this cancer. A history of diagnostic and therapeutic x-rays was obtained to investigate the suggested link between radiation exposure and increased risk of myeloma.

Several occupational exposures have been suggested as risk factors for multiple myeloma, mainly from mortality studies on specific occupational groups. To confirm these associations, information about all jobs which the subjects held six months or longer since age 16 was obtained. In addition, a separate section on farm exposures (e.g., type of farming, insecticides) was included since farming has been reported as a risk factor in previous studies.

From the analysis of the questionnaire data, we plan to address some of these suggested findings, evaluate the effects of lifestyle factors on the incidence of multiple myeloma, and determine the factors responsible for the black-white differences in the incidence of this cancer.

RESULTS AND DISCUSSION

Because data analysis is currently underway, results concerning race-specific risk factors for multiple myeloma are not yet available. However, our preliminary findings concerning participation rates may help other researchers planning to investigate the etiology of multiple myeloma.

Among our cases, black females had the highest interview response rates (75%), followed by white females (64%), white males (63%), and black males (58%). The low response rate among black male cases was primarily due to an exceptionally high percentage of these subjects dying prior to interview. Approximately 15% of the cases were either too ill to be interviewed or refused to participate in the study.

Among the controls, the interview response rates (taking into account the response rate to the RDD phase) were highest for black and white females (73%) followed by black males (72%), and white males (68%). The refusal rates were higher among whites than blacks, regardless of gender.

The overall response rates to the blood collection phase of the study took into account both the interview response rates of those subjects preselected to be included in the blood collection phase and the response to the blood component only. The low interview response rates of the male cases, mainly due to the high death rate, had a substantial impact on the overall blood collection participation rate. This rate, approximately 30%, was similar for both black and white cases. On the other hand, the overall blood collection participation rates for the controls were 48% and 40%, for blacks and whites, respectively.

Among the interviewed subjects asked to participate in the blood component of the study, white controls had the highest refusal rates (33%), followed by black controls (26%), white cases (22%) and black cases (17%). Several factors may have contributed to these refusal rates. Blood drawing was not done at the same time as the interview questionnaire. Thus it was easier for subjects to refuse to participate in the biochemical component over the phone when the phlebotomist attempted to schedule an appointment. Also, the threat of AIDS concerned many subjects. Even after it was explained that there was no risk of contracting AIDS from the procedures, most of these subjects could not be convinced to participate.

In spite of lower-than-anticipated response rates and the complexities in designing and conducting this study, our questionnaire and HLA findings should provide the research community with new insights into the etiology of multiple myeloma among blacks and whites.

Race and Socioeconomic Status Differences in Multiple Myeloma Survival

C.S. Glover, J. Horm, and G. Christenson

Special Populations Studies Branch, National Cancer Institute, National Institutes of Health, Bethesda, MD 20892

ABSTRACT

A study was conducted to investigate black/white differences in the relationship of income and education to survival among patients with multiple myeloma. Five-year relative survival rates were examined for 435 black cases and 1,078 white cases, from three metropolitan areas of the U.S., diagnosed between 1978-1982. In general, survival rates increased as income level increased with blacks experiencing better survival than whites. However, for blacks living in census tracts with the lowest median education level, the survival rates were poorer than the rates for whites. Statistically significant differences in the five-year relative survival rates between blacks and whites were found only in census tracts where the median education level was completion of high school and the median income was at least $15,000 (33.9 and 23.1, respectively, p=.1), and for total income (32.3 and 23.3, respectively, p=.1).

INTRODUCTION

Multiple Myeloma, a malignant neoplasm of plasma cells arising in the bone marrow, is the most common form of monoclonal gammopathy. A common presenting complaint of multiple myeloma is bone pain or pathologic fracture. The cancer is confirmed by radiographic evidence of bone destruction (Pottern 1985). Treatment for multiple myeloma is usually given to control progression or to control symptoms rather than cure the cancer. Chemotherapy and radiation therapy are the primary treatments given for this cancer (Lenhard 1987; Oken 1984) which affects mostly older people. The median age at diagnosis for multiple myeloma is 70 years (National Cancer Institute 1990).

During the past fifteen years, incidence and mortality rates for multiple myeloma have remained stable (National Cancer Institute 1990). Although a rare cancer of low incidence (Table 1), the average annual age-adjusted incidence rate for multiple myeloma, between 1978-1982, for blacks was twice that of whites (7.6 compared to 3.0 cases per 100,000 persons). During that five-year period, black males had the highest incidence of the cancer per 100,000 persons (8.7) followed by black females (6.4), white males (3.5) and white females (2.7). Incidence rates were relatively constant within education and income strata for each race and sex during this period.

The five-year relative survival rate for multiple myeloma patients is poor (Table 2). However, multiple myeloma is one cancer for

Table 1. Average annual age-adjusted incidence rates for multiple myeloma by sex, race, education and income. San Francisco, Atlanta and Detroit metropolitan areas: 1978 - 1982

	Both Sexes		Male		Female	
	White	Black	White	Black	White	Black
			Total Income			
All	3.02	7.55	3.51	8.73	2.68	6.35
Under 12 years	3.63	7.11	4.48	8.62	3.15	5.96
High School	3.24	7.98	3.69	9.22	2.88	6.55
Attended College	2.65	6.70	3.14	6.94	2.32	6.48
			Less than $15,000			
All	3.90	7.42	4.70	9.22	3.68	5.96
Under 12 years	4.53	6.82	4.55	8.53	5.09	5.55
High School	2.69	7.39	2.91	9.76	2.77	5.56
Attended College	5.75	27.66	9.41	17.12	3.02	32.56
			$15,000 and Over			
All	2.99	7.68	3.46	8.28	2.64	6.75
Under 12 years	3.34	9.69	4.46	9.38	2.52	9.72
High School	3.25	8.32	3.72	8.91	2.89	7.11
Attended College	2.59	5.18	3.01	6.14	2.31	4.73

Note: Rates are per 100,000 persons in the population.

which the five-year relative survival rate for blacks has been reported to be higher (National Cancer Institute 1988) than for whites (28.6 percent compared to 25.8 percent between 1978-1982). While race alone has not been shown to be a significant factor in multiple myeloma survival (Alexanian 1975; Savage 1984), several studies have shown low socioeconomic status (SES) to be associated with poorer survival from diseases in general (Berg 1977; California Tumor Registry 1963; Kaplan 1987; Lipworth 1970; Page 1980). A few studies have shown a relationship between the prognosis of multiple myeloma and factors associated with SES. In one such study, patients living in block groups with overcrowding in the home were found to have experienced significantly lower survival rates for multiple myeloma than patients living in block groups with no overcrowding (Savage 1984). In another study, investigators concluded that the ability of multiple myeloma patients to travel a distance to receive health care was related to having better resources and a better prognosis (Lenhard 1987). In a third study of multiple myeloma patients at the University of Iowa Hospitals between 1940-1969, the five-year crude survival rate for indigent patients was 50 percent lower than the rate for private patients (Berg 1977).

Table 2. Five-year relative survival rates for multiple myeloma by sex, race, education and income. San Francisco, Atlanta and Detroit metropolitan areas: 1978 - 1982

	Both Sexes		Male		Female	
	White	Black	White	Black	White	Black
			Total Income			
All	25.8	28.6	25.4	24.0	26.1	33.3
Under 12 years	27.2	20.3	25.2	14.6	29.1	26.3
High School	23.3*	32.3*	20.3	27.3	26.1	37.3
Attended College	30.2	45.4	35.5	-	25.4	-
			Less than $15,000			
All	21.3	25.1	22.2	18.7	20.6	32.9
Under 12 years	15.2	19.9	-	13.1	-	27.5
High School	27.8	29.8	-	23.0	-	39.3
Attended College	-	-	-	-	-	-
			$15,000 and Over			
All	26.1	33.0	25.6	32.1	26.5	33.7
Under 12 years	33.8	-	28.2	-	40.0	-
High School	23.1*	33.9*	20.4	30.8	25.6	36.3
Attended College	30.3	-	35.1	-	26.0	-

- Observed number of cases was too small to do valid survival analyses.
* The difference in rates between blacks and whites is statistically significant (p=.1).

Note: Survival rates are relative rates expressed as percents.

METHODS

Multiple Myeloma cases from the metropolitan areas of Atlanta, San Francisco and Detroit were used for this report. These three areas were used because they have population based tumor registries and black populations large enough to do black/white comparisons, and they are census tracted. The five-year relative survival rates reported here were based on 435 cases for blacks (226 males and 209 females) and 1,078 cases for whites (536 males and 542 females), diagnosed between 1978-1982 (Table 3). Because Atlanta, San Francisco and Detroit metropolitan areas consist solely of urban populations, the results described here may not be representative of the entire U.S. population.

To examine the relationship of SES factors to black/white differences in multiple myeloma survival rates, the proxy SES measures of census tract median family income and median years of education completed were used. Median family income was stratified into two groups: Less than $15,000; and at least $15,000. These two strata were selected to ensure enough cases for meaningful analyses (Table 3).

Three median education levels were compared: Under twelve years; completion of high school; and at least attended college.

Survival rates were tested at the .10 level using 90% confidence intervals. None of the survival rates were significant at the .05 level.

RESULTS

In general, the survival rate trend for both blacks and whites increased as education and income levels increased. However, there was a decrease in survival rates for whites living in census tracts where completion of high school was the median education level. Although not statistically significant, the overall five-year relative survival rates for blacks with multiple myeloma were generally higher than the rates for whites (Table 2). Similar trends existed within most education and income strata.

Survival rates for blacks living in census tracts where the median education level was less than twelve years of school were lower than those rates for whites, although these data were not statistically significant. The survival rates for whites and blacks were 27.2 percent and 20.3 percent, respectively (Table 2).

Table 3. Number of multiple myeloma cases by sex, race, education and income. San Francisco, Atlanta, and Detroit metropolitan areas: 1978 - 1982

	Both Sexes		Male		Female	
	White	Black	White	Black	White	Black
			Total Income			
All	1,078	435	536	226	542	209
Under 12 years	90	169	45	90	45	79
High School	643	238	321	123	322	115
Attended College	345	28	170	13	175	15
			Less than $15,000			
All	73	248	35	139	38	109
Under 12 years	34	147	15	80	19	67
High School	26	94	13	56	13	38
Attended College	13	7	7	3	6	4
			$15,000 and Over			
All	1,005	187	501	87	504	100
Under 12 years	56	22	30	10	26	12
High School	617	144	308	67	309	77
Attended College	332	21	163	10	169	11

Survival rates for blacks and whites living in census tracts with a median income less than $15,000 were similar although rates for blacks were slightly higher. The five-year relative survival rate for blacks living in census tracts where the median income was at least $15,000 and median education level was completion of high school was significantly better than those for whites (33.9 percent compared to 23.1 percent, p=.1).

The difference in survival rates between whites and blacks is largely attributable to the higher five-year relative survival rate for black females. Black females had higher survival rates than white females for virtually all income and education levels where comparisons could be made. However, white females living in census tracts where the median education level was less than twelve years of school had a survival rate of 29.1 percent compared to black females with a rate of 26.3 percent. As with males, the rates reversed as the education level increased for females. Black females living in census tracts where the median education level was completion of high school had a survival rate of 37.3 percent compared to 26.1 percent for white females.

DISCUSSION

The black/white differences in overall survival rates reported here were not statistically significant. However, a trend towards a more positive prognosis for black multiple myeloma patients when compared to white patients does appear to exist. For those blacks living in census tracts where the median education level was reported as completion of high school or more, this trend of more favorable survival rates was particularly apparent. However, for blacks living in census tracts where the median education level was less than twelve years of school, survival rates were much lower than for whites. This apparent exception is due to the differences in the distribution of black and white cancer cases by income. Rates for black females were also lower than rates for white females in the lowest education level.

Multiple Myeloma outcome appears to be influenced by both race and SES (income and education level). It appears that blacks who are better off economically contribute primarily significantly to the better multiple myeloma survival rates which blacks experience compared to whites. For both blacks and whites, as income level increased survival rates generally increased.

The limited number of cases, particularly for blacks, used in these analyses restrict the conclusions we can draw from these data. However, the existing trends are interesting and with increased numbers of black multiple myeloma cancer cases these analyses can be replicated with increased power. Also, results from the 1990 Decennial Census will provide additional census tract SES data for use in future analyses of multiple myeloma.

REFERENCES

Alexanian R, Balcerzak S, Bonnet J, Gehan E, Haut A, Hewlett J, Monto R (1975) Prognostic factors in multiple myeloma. Cancer 36:1192-1201

Berg JW, Ross R, Latourette HB (1977) Economic status and survival of patients. Cancer 39:467-477

California Tumor Registry (1963) Cancer registration and survival in California. State of California Department of Public Health Berkeley

Kaplan GA, Haan MN, Syme SL, Minkler M, Winkleby M (1987) Socio-economic status and health. In: Amler RW, Dull HB (eds) Closing the gap: The burden of unnecessary illness. University Press, Oxford, New York, p 125

Lenhard RE, Enterline JP, Crowley J, Ho GY (1987) The effects of distance from primary treatment centers on survival among patients with multiple myeloma. J Clin Oncol 5(10):1640-1645

Lipworth L, Abelin T, Connelly RR (1970) Socio-economic factors in the prognosis of cancer patients. J Chronic Dis 23:105-115

National Cancer Institute (1988) 1987 annual cancer statistics review: Including cancer trends: 1950-1985

National Cancer Institute (1990) Cancer statistics review 1973-1987

Oken MM, Tsiatis A, Abramson N, et al (1984) Comparison of standard (MP) with intensive (VBMCP) therapy for the treatment of multiple myeloma. Proc Am Soc Clin Oncol 3:279 (Abstract)

Page WF, Kuntz AJ (1980) Racial and socioeconomic factors in cancer survival. Cancer 45:1029-1040

Pottern LM, Blattner WA (1985) Etiology and epidemiology of multiple myeloma and related disorders. In: Wiernik PH, Canellos GP, Kyle RA, Schiffer CA (eds) Neoplastic disease of the blood. Churchhill Livingstone, New York, p 413

Savage D, Lindenbaum J, Ryzin J, Struening E, Garrett TJ (1984) Race, poverty, and survival in multiple myeloma. Cancer 54:3085-3094

Use of Veterans Administration Data to Identify Possible Risk Factors for Multiple Myeloma among Blacks and Whites

Andrew Z. Keller

Andrew Z. Keller & Associates, 36 Madison Street N.E
Washington, D.C. 20011

INTRODUCTION

This case-control study's objective is to investigate some factors which may explain the inordinately higher risks of multiple myeloma for black males than for white males (MacMahon 1956; McPherdran 1972; Keller 1975; Cutler 1975). To achieve this objective, use is made of the nation-wide data resources of the Veterans Administration.

MATERIALS AND METHODS

Information was requested (from the nation-wide complex of some 170 United States Veterans Administration Hospitals) on each black and white male with a hospital discharge diagnosis of multiple myeloma, as identified by the International Classification of Disease Rubric 203 (ICD 1968). When identified by this rubric (from January 1, 1970 thru December 31, 1974) a patient was selected if his terminal social security number digit were a 0, 1, 5 or a 9. This procedure yielded a 40% systematic sample of males diagnosed to have multiple myeloma.

In turn, 989 patients were identified from a listing with 13 duplicates. For each of the 976 individual patients, clinical and administrative records were requested from the hospitals. Records were not found for 13 patients and none was received for 19 others. Records were received for 944 (or 96.72%) of the individual patients among whom 150 did not meet the study criteria.

The study criteria include: an histologic diagnosis of definite multiple myeloma, or an histologic diagnosis of probable multiple myeloma, as supported by the description of a specimen in which at least 20% of the cells were plasma cells or 10% had numerous morphologically abnormal forms. But, in the absence of histologic evidence, there combinedly exist osteolytic bone lesions (with or without pathologic fractures) and monoclonal protein either in the serum or in the urine as evidenced by electrophoresis or Bence-Jones urinalysis, (MacMahon 1956; Paredes 1980). Neither bone lesions nor protein abnormalities alone were sufficient evidence to include a person as a case.

The study criteria were met by 794 male patients. These included four residents of Puerto Rico who were excluded from the study. Among the remaining patients were 590 with multiple myeloma newly diagnosed in the study period. Of these, 187 were black and 403 were white. But 12 blacks and 48 whites were diagnosed to have myeloma undisseminated or plasmacytoma. The 60 plasmacytoma patients were also excluded from the study which ultimately comprised 175 black males and 355 white males with multiple myeloma newly diagnosed in the study period.

A control, for each case, was randomly selected from a sequential numerical listing of social security numbers for the 21,424 patients who constituted a 1% sample of male discharges from Veterans Administration Hospitals during the study period. Each control matched its case on sex, race, age (within five years) and type of patient. The patient types were General Medical and Surgical (96.60%), Psychiatric (1.70%), Neurological (1.13%) and Tuberculosis (0.57%). Excluded as controls were patients with cancer of osteogenic, lymphoid or hematopoietic tissues and with fractures or lytic lesions of bone.

Records of cases and controls were abstracted for demographic data on sex, race, religion, marital status, occupations, birthplace, residence and dates (of birth, hospitalizations, and last known vital status), and for clinical data on osteogenic pathology, cancer, admission diagnoses, and on such diagnostic procedures as histological findings, urinalysis, and electrophoresis of serum protein.

The 530 cases were characterized on age. And, for each race, Age Specific Standardized Morbidity Ratios (SMR's) and their 95% Confidence Limits were determined (Mantel 1959; Rothman 1979).

In the SMR's numerators, are the cases observed with multiple myeloma and in their denominators are the cases expected to have multiple myeloma. At risk of this disease were 561,427 white and 114,441 black males. Each of whom was discharged, in 1970, from a Veterans Administration Hospital in the United States (Keller 1975). Within an age interval, the number of cases expected to have multiple myeloma equals the total cases observed times all patients of a given race at risk of the disease divided by the total patients of both races at risk of multiple myeloma in that same age interval.

Determined for each race were relative frequencies, odds ratios and 95% confidence limits of risk factors when a subject was first admitted to a veterans hospital. The risk factors include religious preferences, marital status, geographical attributes and occupational status. The latter is based on the United States Bureau of Census Classification Index of Industries and Occupations in 1970 (U.S. 1971). Geographical attributes comprise birthplace, home residence and ones native residence (i.e.residence in ones birthplace).

Discordant pair data were employed to estimate odds ratios, to estimate tests of significance (with a continuity corrected X^2) and to approximate 95% confidence limits (Breslow 1980). Hence, in testing the null hypothesis, McNemar's test for equality of proportions in matched samples was utilized and confidence limits were computed from tail probabilities of the binomial distribution. Statistical significance is accepted to be at the 5% level.

RESULTS

Presented in table 1, within age groups by race, are the observed and the expected number of multiple myeloma cases with corresponding Standardized Morbidity Ratios (SMR's) and their 95% confidence limits Expected numbers are adjusted to the age distributions of all black and white male patients, at risk of multiple myeloma, when discharged in 1970 from Veterans Administration Hospitals (Keller 1975). The SMR's are markedly higher for blacks than for whites, except below age 45 years when for each race SMR's are similar. The overall SMR of multiple myeloma is 2.86 folds greater for blacks than for whites.

On age, black cases range from 35 to 86 years and white cases range from 27 to 90 years. Median ages are 63.7 years for blacks and 62.7 years for whites. And each race is bimodally distributed on age.

Table 1. Standardized Morbidity Ratios of Multiple Myeloma, with Cases Observed and Expected, by Age and Race

Risk Factors of Age (Years)	Race (Males)	Multiple Myeloma Cases Observed*	Expected^	SMR of MM Obs./Exp. Ratio	95% CL Range
<45	Black	7	5.345	1.31	0.68 to 2.52
<45	White	18	19.655	0.92	0.74 to 1.13
45-54	Black	37	17.663	2.10	1.57 to 2.80
45-54	White	69	88.337	0.79	0.71 to 0.86
55-64	Black	51	24.906	2.05	1.60 to 2.62
55-64	White	115	141.094	0.82	0.76 to 0.88
65+	Black	80	29.970	2.67	2.19 to 3.21
65+	White	153	203.030	0.75	0.71 to 0.80
All Ages	Black	175	77.884	2.25	1.95 to 2.59
All Ages	White	355	452.116	0.79	0.75 to 0.82

SMR: Standardized Morbidity Ratios
CL: Confidence Limits
MM: Multiple Myeloma

*: The observed cases comprise a 40% systematic sample of black and white males with MM newly diagnosed in a 5-year period when discharged, from U.S. Veterans Administration Hospitals.

^: In an age interval, the cases expected are [(all cases observed to have MM) times (all patients of a given race at risk of MM)] divided by (all patients at risk of MM). Age specific SMR's are determined in reference to 114,441 black and 561,427 white male at risk of MM during 1970 in Veterans Hospitals (Keller 1975).

Shown in table 2 are the religious preferences and marital status of case-control pairs, by race, with corresponding relative frequencies, odds ratios and 95% confidence limits. Most subjects are Protestants. Catholics and Jews are more common among whites. However, case-control pair distributions are similar for each race.

By marital status, only among blacks are case-control pairs similarly distributed. Among whites, the odds ratio is significantly low for persons either single or divorced and is significantly high for persons widowed.

Distributed in table 3 are some geographical attributes of multiple myeloma case-control pairs. Blacks were principally born in the South Most whites were born in the North. Yet, among whites born outside of the U.S., MM cases are significantly excessive. Even so, by place of residence, case-control pairs for each race are similarly distributed despite a marked deficit of white resident cases in the North.

Native residence, seen also in table 3, is residence in the region of one's birth. Native black residents with multiple myeloma are markedly excessive in the South in contrast to either the North solely or the joint regions of the North and West. Yet, for whites, native residence appears not to select on their having an inordinate risk of multiple myeloma, despite a marginally high risk of MM among native white residents of the South.

Table 2. Religious Preference and Marital Status of Black and White Male Multiple Myeloma Cases and Their Matched Controls

Factor of	Relative Percent Cases	Relative Percent Controls	Odds Ratio and 95% C.L. Value	Lower	Upper
A. Religious Preference among 175 Black Pairs					
Protestants	90.9	90.9	1.00	0.42	2.39
Catholics	8.6	9.1	0.93	0.38	2.25
Not Stated	0.5	0.0	NC	----	----
B. Religious Preference among 355 White Pairs					
Protestants	70.4	72.4	0.90	0.61	1.31
Catholics	23.1	23.1	1.00	0.68	1.48
Jews	2.0	2.3	0.88	0.25	3.03
Others/NS	4.5	2.2	2.00	0.75	5.71
C. Marital Status among 175 Black Pairs					
Married	70.9	68.0	1.15	0.69	1.91
Single	8.6	10.9	0.78	0.34	1.74
Divorced	9.1	12.0	0.75	0.34	1.62
Widowed	11.4	9.1	1.27	0.58	2.79
D. Marital Status among 355 White Pairs					
Married	74.1	68.2	1.36	0.94	1.95
Single	9.6	15.2	0.58*	0.34	0.97
Divorced	6.7	11.5	0.54*	0.29	0.99
Widowed	9.6	5.1	2.23**	1.06	4.83

Case-control pairs are matched on sex, race, age (within 5-years) and type of patient, i.e. General Medical and Surgical, Neurological, Psychiatric and Tuberculosis.

C.L.: Confidence Limits
NC: Non-calculable   NS: Not Stated
*: $p < 0.035$ **: $p \leq 0.025$

Table 3. Geographical Attributes of Black and White Male Multiple Myeloma Cases and Their Matched Controls

Geography by	Relative Percent Cases	Controls	Odds Ratio and 95% C.L. Value	Lower	Upper
A. Region of Birth among 175 Black Pairs					
North	10.3	7.4	1.42	0.60	3.41
South	88.6	90.9	0.78	0.34	1.74
Other#	1.1	1.7	0.67	0.04	7.50
B. Region of Birth among 355 White Pairs					
North	45.6	54.1	0.65**	0.44	0.95
South	39.1	38.3	1.06	0.70	1.61
West	7.3	4.4	1.83	0.81	4.23
Outside of U.S.	7.0	3.1	2.56**	1.06	6.54
C. Region of Residence among 175 Black Pairs					
North	34.3	36.0	0.92	0.55	1.54
South	57.7	53.1	1.22	0.75	1.97
West	8.0	10.9	0.64	0.23	1.72
D. Region of Residence among 355 White Pairs					
North	42.0	51.6	0.55^	0.36	0.83
South	39.1	33.8	1.45	0.95	2.24
West	18.9	14.6	1.48	0.90	2.47
E. Native Residence among 109 Black Pairs					
North	13.8	32.1	0.33^	0.14	0.75
South	84.4	56.0	4.10^^	1.89	9.45
West	1.8	11.9	NC	----	----
(North & West)	(15.6)	(44.0)	(0.24)^^	(0.11)	(0.53)
F. Native Residence among 239 White Pairs					
North	46.4	51.4	0.69	0.40	1.20
South	44.4	37.7	1.62	0.94	2.80
West	9.2	10.9	0.79	0.36	1.72

Case-control pairs are matched on sex, race, age (within 5-years) and patient type, i.e. General Medical and Surgical, Neurological, Psychiatric and Tuberculosis.

C.L.: Confidence Limits
Other#: The West and Outside of the U.S.
NC: Non-calculable

**: $p \leq 0.025$ ^: $p < 0.005$ ^^: $p < 0.0005$

Seen in table 4 is the occupational status of case-control pairs by race. When blacks and whites are compared, as either cases or controls, their distributions differ significantly on occupations. In both races, persons unemployed or retired have remarkably low risks of multiple myeloma. Among blacks, while multiple myeloma risks are indeed high for professionals, managers, craftsmen and farmers, the disease risk is significantly high only for craftsmen. Among whites, however, no occupational category is associated with an inordinately high risk of multiple myeloma.

Table 4. Occupational Status of Black and White Male Multiple Myeloma Cases and Their Matched Controls

Occupational Status of	Relative Percent Cases	Controls	Odds Ratio and 95% C.L. Value	Lower	Upper
A. 175 Black Male Pairs					
Profs. & Mgrs.	5.1	2.9	1.80	0.48	7.53
Clericals & Sales	4.0	8.5	0.43	0.13	1.31
Craftsmen	18.3	9.7	2.07*	1.01	4.38
Operatives	20.0	19.4	1.04	0.57	1.91
Farmers	11.4	6.3	1.82	0.78	4.38
Svc. Wrks.	25.7	18.9	1.60	0.85	3.03
Laborers	14.3	24.0	0.50**	0.25	0.96
Unemp./Others	1.2	10.3	0.11^^	0.09	0.56
B. 355 White Male Pairs					
Profs. & Mgrs.	12.7	9.6	1.36	0.81	2.28
Clericals & Sales	11.6	9.6	1.24	0.72	2.15
Craftsmen	27.6	26.2	1.07	0.75	1.51
Operatives	20.8	14.9	1.47	0.97	2.22
Farmers	9.3	11.0	0.83	0.48	1.43
Svc. Wrks.	8.7	11.3	0.75	0.43	1.31
Laborers	7.0	10.1	0.69	0.38	1.23
Unemployed	1.4	4.2	0.29*	0.06	1.04
Others	0.9	3.1	0.27	0.04	1.21
(Unemp./Others)	(2.3)	(7.3)	(0.28)*	(0.10)	(0.73)

Case-control pairs are matched on sex, race, age (within five-years) and type of patient (i.e. General Medical and Surgical, Neurological, Psychiatric and Tuberculosis).

C.L.: Confidence Limits
Profs. & Mgrs.: Professionals and Managerials
Svc. Wrks.: Service Workers
Unemp./Others: Unemployed/Retired or Not Stated

*: $p < 0.035$ **: $p \leq 0.025$ ^^: $p < 0.0005$

DISCUSSION

This study's objective is to investigate marital status, religious preferences, geography, occupations and age as possible risk factors which may contribute to explain the inordinately higher risks of multiple myeloma for black than for white males (MacMahon 1956; McPherdran 1972; Keller 1975; Cutler 1975; Blattner 1980; Young 1981).

The 530 cases, in this study, constitute a 40% systematic sample of black and white males with multiple myeloma newly diagnosed in a five year period. Each case was identified by the International Classification of Disease Rubric 203 and was confirmed on the basis of elaborate diagnostic criteria (MacMahon 1956; Paredes 1980). A control, for each case, was randomly selected and matched to its case on race, age (within 5-years), and patient type.

All study subjects resided in contiguous States of the U.S. and the District of Columbia. Each was similarly selected for hospitalization on the basis of a service-connected disability and the ability to pay for medical care. Each subject was similarly treated at and discharged from Veterans Administration Hospitals (where all records are uniformly indexed) between January 1, 1970 and December 31, 1974.

It was found that the overall Standardized Morbidity Ratio of multiple myeloma is 2.86 folds greater for blacks than for whites. And, except for ages below 45 years, the Age Specific Standardized Morbidity Ratio's are significantly higher for blacks. For each race, the median ages are similar and the age distributions are bimodally distributed. This age bimodality is due to the effects of war time military services on the base veterans population from which veterans in civil life were selected for hospitalization.

It is notable that the base veterans' population (within the case's age range) constitutes 50.8% of the entire United States male population. However, findings in the present study apply most aptly to veterans discharged from Veterans Administration Hospitals in the U.S.

When compared with their matched controls, the widowed whites have a significantly high risk of multiple myeloma, as do whites foreign-born particularly in Canada and Europe. These foreign born whites reside mainly in the North and South where, for them, the risk of multiple myeloma is 2.83 folds higher than for other whites. Also, this disease risk is significantly high for black native residents of the South and black craftsmen. There also exists a markedly low multiple myeloma risk: 1) For whites who are single, divorced, born or resident in the North, or unemployed, and; 2) For blacks who are laborers, unemployed or native residents of the North.

By occupations, as either cases or controls, whites are distributed significantly different than corresponding blacks. These differences are typified by whites, unlike blacks, being employed mainly as white collar workers and craftsmen but not as laborers and service workers. Moreover, in many studies other than this one, farming (among whites) is reportedly associated with significantly high risks of multiple myeloma (Milham 1971; Gallagher 1983; Pearce 1986; Linet 1987; Cantor 1984; Brownson 1988).

Most findings, in this study, appear to have no definitive biological basis. Yet many do suggest that life style (in relation to marital status) and environmental exposures (in association with employment, birthplace and residence) may contribute to explain why blacks often have inordinately different risks than whites of multiple myeloma. Even so, future analyses of these and similar data on multiple myeloma should employ multivariate techniques.

Acknowledgements: The author is grateful for the support of the Veterans Administration's Department of Medicine and Surgery which provided these data during his tenure as its Chief of Epidemiologic Research. And, he deeply appreciates Andrew Z. Keller and Associates' President Mrs. Frances Carmicheal Keller and Manager Mr. Lord Brazil Waters for their commitments to this research endeavor.

REFERENCES

1. Blattner W (1980) Epidemiology of Multiple Myeloma and Related Plasma Cell Disorders: An Analytic Review. In: Potter ed. Progress in Myeloma. Elsevier North Holland, Inc., NY, pp 1-65

2. Breslow NE, Day NE (1980) Statistical Methods In Cancer Research Vol.I-The Analysis of Case-Control Studies. International Agency for Research on Cancer, Lyon, pp 162-189

3. Brownson RC, Reif JS (1988) A cancer registry-based study of occupational risk for lymphoma, multiple myeloma and leukaemia. Int J Epidemiol 17:27-32

4. Cantor KP, Blair A (1984) Farming and mortality from multiple myeloma: A case-control study with the use of death certificates. J Natl Cancer Inst 72:251-255

5. Cutler SJ, Young JL (1975) The Third National Cancer Survey: Incidence Data. Natl Cancer Inst Monogr 41

6. Gallagher RP, Spinelli JJ, Elwood JM, Skippen DH (1983) Allergies and agricultural exposure as risk factors for multiple myeloma. Br J Cancer 48:853-857

7. International Classification of Diseases, Eight Revision, Adapted for use in the United States-Vol I. (1968) PHS Publ No. 1693. U.S. Government Printing Office, Washington, D.C.,pp 121-123

8. Keller AZ (1975) Morbidity Patterns of Cancer in the United States. In: The Society for Epidemiologic Research's Abstracts on Malignant Neoplasms in Hospitals. Amer J Epidemiol 102:450-452

9. Linet MS, Harlow SD, McLaughlin JK (1987) A case-control study of multiple myeloma in whites: chronic antigenic stimulation, occupation and drug use. Cancer Res 47:2978-2981

10. MacMahon B, Clark DW (1956) The Incidence of Multiple Myeloma. J Chron Dis 4:508-515

11. Mantel N, Haenszel W (1959) Statistical Aspects of the Analyses of Data from Retrospective Studies of Disease. JNCI 22:719-748

12. McPherdran P, Heath CW Jr., Garcia J (1972) Multiple Myeloma Incidence in Metropolitan Atlanta, Ga.: Racial and Seasonal Variations. Blood 39:866-873

13. Milham A Jr (1971) Leukemia and Multiple Myeloma in Farmers. Am J Epidemiol 94:307-310

14. Rothman KJ, Boice, JD Jr (1979) Epidemiologic analysis with a programmable calculator. Washington, DC: U.S. Government Printing Office, [(US DHHS (PHS,NIH) NIH publication no. 79-1649)].

15. Paredes JM, Mitchell BS (July 1980) Multiple Myeloma. Med Clin of North America 64(45):743-760

16. Pearce NE, Smith AH, Howard JK, et al (1986) Case-control study of multiple myeloma and farming. Br J Cancer 54:493-500.

17. U.S. Bureau of Census, 1970 Census of Population. (1971) "Classification Index of Industries and Occupations." Washington, DC: U.S. Government Printing Office, pp 0-1 to 0-137

18. Young JL, Percy, MS et al (1981) Cancer Incidence and Mortality in the United States, 1973-1977. SEER, NCI Monogr 57, pp 1-187

Multiple Myeloma in Sub-Sahara Africa

Robert J. Jacobson

Georgetown University Medical Center, 3800 Reservoir Road N.W., Washington, D.C. 20007

Multiple myeloma and other plasma cell neoplasms have been minimally reported for the large population living in sub-Sahara Africa. While the incidence of multiple myeloma in black Americans and Jamaicans is considered the highest in the world there are few studies documenting the incidence and clinicopathologic features in blacks from Africa.

Over ten years ago Shulman, Jacobson and Blattner reported in several articles (1974, 1975, 1978, 1979, 1980) the incidence, clinicopathologic and immunochemical features of plasma cell dyscrasias in blacks and whites living in the metropolitan area of Johannesburg South Africa. They noted that the age-adjusted rates (world standard) per 100,000 were 7.47 in black males and 5.11 in black females (1979). These patients were all diagnosed and evaluated in Beragwarath Hospital, Soweto in the two year period 1973 to 1975. In this period multiple myeloma was diagnosed in 29 blacks (19 male and 10 female patients). Comparative age-adjusted rates for Johannesburg white males were 7.84 per 100,000 and 3.34 per 100,000 white females (1979). Prior to this reported high incidence of multiple myeloma it was believed that low rates prevailed in Africa. In large part this was due to underdiagnosis and the lack of medical and laboratory facilities necessary to establish the diagnosis.

In a large series of 123 consecutive patients (49 blacks and 74 whites) observed over a 6 year period - 1971 to 1976 - in Johannesburg, Shulman and Jacobson (1974) and (1980) noted that IgA myeloma occurred relatively more frequently in the blacks than in the white patients. The distribution of the other immunochemical classes was otherwise similar in both race groups. Pathologic fractures often of the thoracolumbar spine were a common clinical feature of the black patients. The median age of clinical presentation in the blacks was 52 years, a decade younger than the median age for the white patients. Solitary plasmacytoma of bone or extramedullary tumors were found in 10 black patients and in only 1 white patient in this 6 (six) year period. In contrast, monoclonal gammopathy of undetermined significance was documented only in white subjects (1974). It is most likely that in the black population medical attention was sought only when individuals became symptomatic. Walderstrom's macroglobulinemia has rarely been reported in sub-Sahara Africa. Shulman and Jacobson documented this disease in 8 black and 10 white patients (1980). Sacher et al (1978) reported the detailed chemopathologic findings in 4 of these patients and other than a young age at presentation (mean 43 years), the features were typical of the disease. Clinical and pathologic descriptions of multiple myeloma have been reported from patients in Central, East and West Africa. Tozer et al (1980) reviewed the experience in Malawi from 1969 to 1978. Twenty-nine cases were diagnosed and 20 of them presented with a large-bone tumor mass and the diagnosis was made histologically from a biopsy specimen. These authors also commented on the problems of diagnostic facilities and the underdiagnosis of this disease in Africa. Waldbaum and Gelfand (1974) described 12 cases from Zimbabwe in 1974 and Levy updated the experience from this country in 1988 (1988). She reported on the relative frequencies of hematologic and lymphoreticular malignancies observed at two central hospitals in Harare over a 3 year period - 1982-1984. She noted 74 cases of multiple myeloma and the relative frequency was 21.3%. Leukemia was diagnosed in 42% and non-Hodgkins lymphoma in 25.7% of patients during this period.

There are typical cases of myeloma documented in Zambia (1977) Uganda (1974) and Kenya (1981). Mukiibi et al (1981) reported in 1981 on patients (20 male, 16 female) in Nairobi, and the mean age was 52.5 years. They later expanded the series (1988) to 75 patients and again noted the mean age at 51 years and stated that the disease appeared to be more prevalent in Kenyan Africans, than previously believed. The younger age of presentation in African patients needs to be viewed against the overall population age distribution. There is a smaller percentage of the African population over 60 years of age, than populations in North America and Europe. A recent paper by Onyemelukwe and Kulkarni (1988), reviewed the experience in Northern Nigeria from 1971 to 1985. There were 24 male patients and 15 female patients and the age range was 35 to 70 years (mean 52 years). In all the series of African patients there is a male predominance, as has been noted elsewhere in the world. Surprisingly in this Nigerian study, the authors reported that 25% of patients had IgM secreting myeloma. Bone pain, especially in the back, was the commonest persisting complaint and 5 patients had collapse of a thoracolumbar vertebra.

It appears that there are pertinent case studies of multiple myeloma in sub-Sahara Africa but epidemiologic information needs to be gathered. From the observations in North America and Jamaica and the findings amongst the Black population in Johannesburg, it could be anticipated that the incidence of myeloma in Africa is significantly greater than what has been reported to date.

REFERENCES

Amsel S, Nabembezi JS (1974) Two year survey of hematologic malignancies in Uganda. J Natl Cancer Inst 52(5):1397-401

Blattner WA, Jacobson RJ, Shulman G (1979) Multiple myeloma in South African Blacks. Lancet 1:928-9

Jacobson RJ, Levy JI, Shulman G and De Moor NG (1975) Solitary myeloma. A study of 10 black patients during an 8 year period. S Afr Med J 49:1347-1351

Levy LM (1988) The pattern of haematological and lymphoreticular malignancy in Zimbabwe. Trop Geogr Med 40(2):109-14

Mukiibi JM, Karimi M, Kyobe J (1981) Multiple myeloma in Kenyan Africans - a prospective study. East Afr Med J 58(3):171-80

Mukiibi JM, Kyobe J (1988) Pattern of multiple myeloma in Kenyans. Trop Geogr Med 40(1):20-5

Onyemelukwe GC, Kulkarni AG (1988) Immunoglobulin types and features of multiple myeloma in northern Nigeria. East Afr Med J 65(1):33-8

Sacher RA, Jacobson RJ, Derman D and Shulman G (1978) Waldenstrom's macroglobulinemia in South African Negroes. Trop Geog Med 30-207-214

Shulman G and Jacobson RJ (1980) Immunocytoma in Black and White South Africans. Trop Geog Med 32(2):112-117

Shulman G, Stevens K, Bernard DB et al. (1974) Multiple myeloma: Clinical, biochemical and immunochemical aspects. S Afr Med J 48:1023-1026

Tozer RA, Clear AS, Davies DR, Hutt MS (1980) Unusual presentation of patients with myelomatosis in Malawi. J Clin Pathol, 33(6):544-6

Traub N (1977) Multiple myeloma at the University Teaching Hospital. Med J Zambia 11(5):148-50

Waldbaum B and Gelfand M (1974) Myelomatosis in the Rhodesian Africa. Trop Geogr Med 26:26-30

Monoclonal Gammopathies and Multiple Myeloma

Case Definition: Issues Related to Monoclonal Gammopathies and Multiple Myeloma

Robert A. Kyle, M.D.
Chairman, Division of Hematology and Internal Medicine, Consultant, Division of Laboratory Medicine, Mayo Clinic and Mayo Foundation; Professor of Medicine and of Laboratory Medicine, Mayo Medical School; Rochester, Minnesota 55905

During 1988, 808 patients were found with a serum monoclonal protein (M-protein) at the Mayo Clinic. The most frequent clinical diagnosis was monoclonal gammopathy of undetermined significance (MGUS) (benign monoclonal gammopathy), 64%. Other diagnoses were multiple myeloma (MM), 14%; primary systemic amyloidosis (AL), 8%; lymphoproliferative disease including lymphoma and macroglobulinemia, 8%; chronic lymphocytic leukemia, 2%; smoldering multiple myeloma (SMM), 2%; and solitary or extramedullary plasmacytoma, 2%.

The term MGUS denotes the presence of an M-protein in patients without evidence of multiple myeloma, lymphoproliferative diseases, amyloidosis, or related disorders. The term "benign" monoclonal gammopathy is misleading because one does not know at the time of recognition whether an M-protein will remain stable and benign or whether it represents or develops into symptomatic multiple myeloma, malignant lymphoproliferative disease, or amyloidosis.

MGUS is characterized by a serum level less than 3 g/dL, fewer than 5% plasma cells in the bone marrow, none or only small amounts of M-protein in the urine, absence of lytic bone lesions, anemia, hypercalcemia, and renal insufficiency, and, most importantly, stability of the M-protein and failure of development of other abnormalities. Approximately 3% of patients older than 70 years and 1% of those older than 50 years have a serum M-protein without evidence of multiple myeloma, macroglobulinemia, amyloidosis, or related diseases (Axelsson 1966; Kyle 1972; Saleun 1982).

The incidence of monoclonal gammopathies increases with advancing age. In Finistère, France, 4% of 720 patients older than 80 years had an M-protein (Saleun 1982). In another study utilizing agarose gel electrophoresis, M-proteins were found in 11 (10%) of 111 patients older than 80 years in a population of ambulatory residents of a retirement home.

In our past experience and that of others, approximately 15% of monoclonal proteins are of the IgM type. In contrast, in a study of 4,193 patients with monoclonal gammopathies from three regions in France, Hurez et al. (1985) reported that 33% were IgM. There is no explanation for this unexpectedly high frequency of IgM.

More sensitive techniques will detect a greater number of M-proteins. For example, Papadopoulos et al. (1982) detected homogeneous bands in the sera of 30 (5%) of 600 healthy adults who were 22 to 65 years of age. Immunoisoelectric focusing, a more sensitive technique, detected an M-protein in the sera of 11% of patients older than 45 years who were hospitalized for surgery of a nonmalignant condition. Agarose electrophoresis detected an M-protein in only 2% of that population (Sinclair 1986).

MAYO CLINIC STUDY

It is of great importance to both the patient and the physician to determine whether an apparently benign monoclonal gammopathy will remain stable or progress to a serious plasma cell proliferative process. We reviewed the medical records of all patients with a monoclonal gammopathy seen at the Mayo Clinic before Jan. 1, 1971. Patients with multiple myeloma, macroglobulinemia, amyloidosis, lymphoma, or related disorders were excluded. Two hundred forty-one patients remained for long-term study.

Four percent were younger than 40 years and one-third were 70 years or older when the M-protein was recognized. The median age of the patients was 64 years.

The liver was palpable in 15% of patients, and the spleen was palpable in 4%. In those with hepatosplenomegaly 5 cm or more below the costal margin, the causes were congestive heart failure, myelofibrosis with myeloid metaplasia, cirrhosis, or other conditions not directly related to the monoclonal gammopathy.

Anemia was not a feature of the monoclonal gammopathy. In the nine patients whose hemoglobin value was less than 10 g/dL, melena, myeloid metaplasia, myeloproliferative disease, Wegener's granulomatosis, hypoplasia of bone marrow, chronic cold agglutinin disese, and hypernephroma were responsible. Five patients had a platelet count less than 100,000/mm^3. The causes included myeloid metaplasia, acute leukemia, idiopathic thrombocytopenic purpura, lupus erythematosus, and hypoplasia of the bone marrow. The serum creatinine value was greater than 2.0 mg/dL in five patients. This was related to nephrosclerosis in three, diabetes mellitus in one, and uric acid nephropathy in one.

The monoclonal protein was IgG in 74%, IgA in 10%, and IgM in 16%. The median size of the M-protein was 1.7 g/dL. The light-chain type was κ in 63% and λ in the remainder. Biclonal gammopathy was present in 2.1%. The heavy-chain class and the light-chain type did not change throughout the period of observation. The uninvolved or background immunoglobulins were reduced in 28% of the group. The subclasses were as follows: IgG1 (86%), IgG2 (4%), IgG3 (4%), and IgG4 (6%).

Fifteen patients had a monoclonal light chain in the urine at the time of recognition of the serum M-protein. Nine were κ and the remainder λ. The M-protein was 1 g or less per 24 hours in all but three patients. The percentage of bone marrow plasma cells ranged from 1% to 10% (median, 3%).

Associated Diseases

Twenty-six percent of the patients had no disease present at the discovery of the serum M-protein. Thirteen percent had cardiovascular or cerebrovascular disease. Unrelated inflammatory disorders including fever of undetermined origin, deep-vein phlebitis, and chronic inflammatory bowel disease were found in 11%. An unrelated malignancy was present in 7%. Neurologic disorders and connective tissue diseases accounted for 6% each. Hematologic disorders including myelofibrosis with myeloid metaplasia, idiopathic thrombocytopenic purpura, von Willebrand's disease, hypoplastic anemia, red cell aplasia, idiopathic neutropenia, and undifferentiated myeloproliferative diseases accounted for 4%. The remainder had a wide variety of disorders that were unrelated to the M-protein.

Findings at Follow-Up of the 241 Patients

<u>Group 1 (Stable; 57 Patients, 24%)</u>: At current follow-up (median, 19 years; range, 11 to 32 years), approximately one-fourth of patients had a stable M-protein and could be classified as having "benign" monoclonal gammopathy (Kyle and Lust, 1989). Seventeen of these patients had been followed for 20 or more years. The M-protein disappeared from the serum in only two patients.

The level of the hemoglobin, size of the serum M-protein, and number of plasma cells in the bone marrow did not differ substantially in this group when compared with the total group. Four patients had a monoclonal light chain in the urine that remained stable. One of these four patients had grade 3 to grade 4 proteinuria for 31 years. The urinary monoclonal κ light-chain excretion was 1.5 g/24 hours and has remained stable for the past 13 years. His serum M-protein level has been approximately 2.6 g/dL for 24 years. Renal failure has not developed. Although these 57 patients have been followed for a median of 19 years, they must continue to be observed because serious disease is still developing.

<u>Group 2 (Increase in M-Protein Only; 7 Patients, 3%)</u>: The M-protein increased to more than 3 g/dL in seven patients, but they did not develop symptomatic multiple myeloma, macroglobulinemia, or other diseases and have not been treated. The range of increase was 1.1 to 2.3 g/dL (median, 1.5 g/dL). The median interval from the recognition of the M-protein to the level of 3.0 g/dL was 11 years. The usual pattern of increase of the M-protein was gradual, but there was waxing and waning of the level.

<u>Group 3 (Died Without Development of Myeloma, Macroglobulinemia, Amyloidosis, or Related Disorders; 124 Patients, 51%)</u>: The median interval from recognition of the M-protein to death was 7.9 years. Thirty-nine percent of the patients survived more than 10 years after the M-protein was found. Fifteen of the 124 patients developed a serum M-protein of 3.0 g/dL or greater during observation, but none had symptomatic multiple myeloma or macroglobulinemia requiring therapy. Cardiac disease was the most frequent cause of death, followed by cerebrovascular disease and malignancy.

<u>Group 4 (Developed Multiple Myeloma, Macroglobulinemia, Amyloidosis, or Related Diseases; 53 Patients, 22%)</u>: The actuarial rate of development of these diseases was 17% at 10 years and 33% at 20 years.

Thirty-six of the 53 patients (68%) developed symptomatic multiple myeloma requiring chemotherapy. All but two patients had a bone marrow aspirate or biopsy that contained more than 15% abnormal plasma cells at the time of diagnosis of multiple myeloma. Of the two exceptions, one had a paravertebral mass with destruction and collapse of T-5 and the other had a large destructive plasmacytoma of the sacrum. Twenty-nine of the 36 patients with myeloma had a serum M-protein level greater than 3 g/dL. Eighteen patients had an M-protein in the urine. Anemia was present in all but four patients. Lytic bone lesions were found in 16 patients, osteoporosis and compression fractures in 3, destructive bone lesions in 2, osteoporosis in 1, and a large extradural plasmacytoma in 1. These findings fulfill the criteria for the diagnosis of multiple myeloma.

The interval from the time of recognition of the monoclonal gammopathy to the diagnosis of multiple myeloma ranged from 23 to 251 months (median, 115 months [9.6 years]). The median survival after the diagnosis of multiple myeloma was 35 months. The myeloma developed either gradually or abruptly. In 19 patients the M-protein was stable for 5 to 21 years, after which multiple myeloma developed abruptly or gradually during periods up to 6 years. In seven other patients, the M-protein was stable for 11 to 41 months before multiple myeloma developed.

Macroglobulinemia of Waldenström developed in seven patients. The median interval from recognition of the M-protein to the diagnosis of macroglobulinemia was 8.5 years. Six of the patients had serum levels of IgMκ monoclonal protein that ranged from 3.1 to 8.5 g/dL during the course of the disease. One patient had a biclonal gammopathy (IgMκ and IgAκ). The bone marrow aspirates or biopsies or autopsy specimens showed increased numbers of lymphocytes and plasma cells in all cases. Anemia was a feature of all seven patients.

Primary systemic amyloidosis (AL) was found in seven patients 6 to 16.5 years after the recognition of the M-protein (median, 8 years). The diagnosis of amyloidosis was based upon tissue obtained at autopsy in three cases, renal biopsy in two, lymph node biopsy in one, and rectal biopsy in one.

The remaining three patients developed a lymphoproliferative disease. One patient presented with a biclonal gammopathy (IgGλ and IgMκ) and lupus erythematosus. An aggressive, diffuse, undifferentiated malignant lymphoma developed 7 years later, and the patient died. Another patient had an IgMλ monoclonal protein for 22 years when she developed anorexia, weight loss, and generalized bone pain. A diagnosis of immunoblastic lymphoma was made on the basis of a bone marrow aspirate and biopsy. Extensive retroperitoneal lymphadenopathy was found on a computed tomography scan. Malignant-appearing lymphocytes were found in the cerebrospinal fluid. The patient did not respond to chemotherapy and died 1 month later. In another patient, chronic lymphocytic leukemia developed after 56 months of observation. Four courses of chlorambucil were given for recurrent lymphocytosis. The IgMκ monoclonal protein remained stable for 16 years and probably was not directly related to the chronic lymphocytic leukemia. The patient died 18.5 years after recognition of the M-protein.

The serum M-protein did not increase in 10 of the 53 patients: 1 with multiple myeloma who had a small monoclonal IgAκ (1.8 g/dL) but a large increase in urinary light chain (0.7 to 3.2 g/24 hours), 6 with amyloidosis, 2 with lymphoma, and 1 with chronic lymphocytic leukemia. Five of the 10 patients had an IgM monoclonal gammopathy.

Analysis by Immunoglobulin Group

The actuarial rate of development of serious disease in the 203 patients with an IgG or an IgA monoclonal protein was 13% at 10 years and 29% at 20 years. The actuarial rate of development of a serious disease in the 38 patients with an IgM monoclonal protein was 21% at 10 years and 49% at 20 years.

In addition, seven patients (3%) had an M-protein value of 3.0 g/dL or more during follow-up but did not develop symptomatic multiple myeloma or other serious disease. Sixty patients who developed a serious plasma cell proliferative process or an M-protein of more than 3 g/dL accounted for 23% of those with IgG or IgA and 37% of those with an IgM monoclonal gammopathy.

DIFFERENTIATION OF MGUS FROM MULTIPLE MYELOMA AND MACROGLOBULINEMIA

Minimal criteria for the diagnosis of multiple myeloma consist of 10% or more abnormal plasma cells in the bone marrow or histologic proof of a plasmacytoma plus one of the following: (1) serum M-protein usually greater than 3 g/dL, (2) M-protein in the urine, or (3) presence of lytic bone lesions. Care must be taken to exclude the possibility of connective tissue diseases, metastatic carcinoma, or other disorders with an unrelated serum M-protein, bone marrow plasmacytosis, or lytic bone lesions.

In addition, one must recognize the subset of patients with smoldering multiple myeloma (SMM). They have a serum M-protein greater than 3 g/dL and more than 10% atypical plasma cells in the bone marrow. Frequently, they have a reduction of uninvolved immunoglobulins in the serum and may have a small monoclonal light chain in the urine. These findings are consistent with multiple myeloma, but anemia, renal insufficiency, and skeletal lesions are not found and the M-protein in the serum and urine and the bone marrow plasma cells remain stable. These patients have a benign monoclonal gammopathy, but it is not possible to make this diagnosis when the patient is initially seen because most patients with this level of M-protein in the serum and urine or bone marrow plasma cells have symptomatic multiple myeloma. Patients with SMM should not be treated unless laboratory abnormalities progress or symptoms of myeloma develop (Kyle 1980).

Differentiation of the patient with benign monoclonal gammopathy from one in whom myeloma or macroglobulinemia eventually develops is very difficult when the M-protein is first recognized. The presence of a serum M-protein of more than 3 g/dL usually indicates overt multiple myeloma or macroglobulinemia, but some exceptions such as SMM exist. In most patients with multiple myeloma, the levels of polyclonal (normal or uninvolved) immunoglobulins are reduced, but a similar reduction may occur in patients with benign monoclonal gammopathy or SMM. The presence of a monoclonal light chain in the urine is suggestive of a neoplastic process, but small amounts of Bence Jones proteinuria may be found in patients with SMM and benign monoclonal gammopathy. The presence of more than 10% plasma cells in the bone marrow is suggestive of multiple myeloma, but some patients with an even greater degree of plasmacytosis have remained stable for long periods. Morphologic features of the plasma cells are of limited use in differentiating benign from malignant disease. The presence of osteolytic lesions suggests multiple myeloma, but metastatic carcinoma may also produce lytic lesions and be associated with an unrelated monoclonal gammopathy.

The plasma cell labeling index measures the synthesis of DNA and is helpful in differentiating the patient with MGUS or SMM from multiple myeloma. An elevated plasma cell labeling index is good evidence that a patient has multiple myeloma or soon will have symptomatic myeloma (Gonchoroff 1985). Levels of β_2-microglobulin, the presence of J chains in malignant plasma cells, or elevated acid phosphatase levels in plasma cells are unreliable for differentiation. Reduced numbers of CD4 T cells, increased numbers of monoclonal idiotype-bearing peripheral lymphocytes, or increased numbers of immunoglobulin-secreting cells in peripheral blood are characteristic of multiple myeloma, but there is overlap with MGUS.

In short, there is no single reliable technique for differentiating a patient with a benign monoclonal gammopathy from one who has or will develop symptomatic multiple myeloma or other malignant disease. The most reliable means of differentiating a benign from a malignant course is the serial measurement of the M-protein in the serum and urine and periodic reevaluation of the clinical and laboratory features to determine whether multiple myeloma, systemic amyloidosis, macroglobulinemia, or other malignant lymphoplasma cell proliferative disorder develops.

REFERENCES

Axelsson U, Bachmann R, Hällen J (1966) Frequency of pathological proteins (M-components) in 6,995 sera from an adult population. Acta Med Scand 179: 235-247

Gonchoroff NJ, Greipp PR, Kyle RA, Katzmann JA (1985) A monoclonal antibody reactive with 5-bromo-deoxyuridine that does not require DNA denaturation. Cytometry 6: 506-512

Hurez D, Youinou P, Gombert J, Preud'homme JL (1985) Survey of monoclonal gammopathy in western France: incidence and unexpected high frequency of IgM. Immunology 56: 557-560

Kyle RA, Greipp PR (1980) Smoldering multiple myeloma. N Engl J Med 302: 1347-1349

Kyle RA, Lust JA (1989) Monoclonal gammopathies of undetermined significance. Semin Hematol 26: 176-200

Kyle RA, Finkelstein S, Elveback LR, Kurland LT (1972) Incidence of monoclonal proteins in a Minnesota community with a cluster of multiple myeloma. Blood 40: 719-724

Papadopoulos NM, Elin RJ, Wilson DM (1982) Incidence of γ-globulin banding in a healthy population by high-resolution electrophoresis. Clin Chem 28: 707-708

Saleun JP, Vicariot M, Deroff P, Morin JF (1982) Monoclonal gammopathies in the adult population of Finistère, France. J Clin Pathol 35: 63-68

Sinclair D, Dagg JH, Dewar AE, Mowat AMcI, Parrott DMV, Stockdill G, Stott DI (1986) The incidence, clonal origin and secretory nature of serum paraproteins in chronic lymphocytic leukaemia. Br J Haematol 64: 725-735

The Frequency of Monoclonal Gammopathy of Unknown Significance in Black and Caucasian Veterans in a Hospital Population

G. P. Schechter, N. Shoff, C. Chan, C. D. McManus, and H. P. Hawley

Veterans Affairs Medical Center and George Washington University, Washington DC, USA

INTRODUCTION

In the United States, for unknown reasons multiple myeloma occurs more frequently in Blacks than Caucasians (Blattner, 1980). To determine whether there is a similar increase of benign paraproteinemia or monoclonal gammopathy of unknown significance (MGUS) (Kyle, 1982) in Blacks, we initiated a screening program at the Washington DC Veterans Affairs Medical Center (Schechter et al, 1986). This study has been extended to include 2721 patients.

METHODS

Sera were obtained from 1877 Black and 859 Caucasian patients who were seen during a 42 month period between 1983 and 1987. There were 2700 males and 36 females, an expected distribution for this hospital's patient population. Most of the serum samples were unselected, obtained from specimens leftover after routine laboratory testing. 535 samples were referred for protein electrophoresis by the patients' physicians. Protein electrophoresis was performed on cellulose acetate. Homogenous bands in the beta and gamma globulin ranges were confirmed as monoclonal by immunofixation on agarose gel. The race of the patients was determined by direct inspection or review of the charts. The age and race of all patients, and the monoclonal immunoglobulin type and level, the non-paraprotein immunoglobulin levels, and the clinical diagnosis of the patients with a paraprotein were entered into a computer file. The majority of the patients were seen by the Hematology consultation service for evaluation for an occult plasma cell or lymphocyte malignancy. Thirteen Black and 2 Caucasian patients with lymphocytic or plasma cell malignancies were excluded, leaving 2721 patients to be evaluated for the frequency of MGUS. The data were analyzed by the Chi-square test.

RESULTS

Eighty-five men and 1 woman, 3.16% of the patients, were found to have MGUS without evidence of multiple myeloma or a lymphoproliferative disorder. Sixty-four patients had monoclonal and 22 patients had biclonal or oligoclonal electrophoretic patterns. There was a significant difference between the percentage of Black and Caucasian patients having paraproteins (3.65% vs 2.10%, X^2 = 4.10, p = 0.043, Table 1).

There were 10 Black patients and no Caucasian patients under the age of 50 who had paraproteinemia. The percentage of patients with MGUS increased with age in both groups, (Blacks, X^2 = 13.74 df 3, p < .01; Caucasians, X^2 = 10.08, p < .05). The distribution of the immunoglobulin types differed in the two groups (Table 2). Seventy-one of 76 (93%) of the paraproteins seen in the Black patients were IgG or

IgA as compared to 10 of 19 (53%) in the white patients ($X^2 = 17.01$, $p < .001$.)

Table 1. Age and Race Distribution of Patients with MGUS

	No. of patients with MGUS/No. screened (%)		
Age	Blacks	Caucasians	Total
≤50 yrs	10/425 (2.35%)	0/135 (0%)	10/560 (1.79%)
51-60 yrs	11/531 (2.07%)	4/218 (1.83%)	15/749 (2.00%)
61-70 yrs	30/648 (4.63%)	5/317 (1.58%)	35/965 (3.63%)
≥71 yrs	17/260 (6.54%)	9/187 (4.81%)	26/447 (5.82%)
Total	68/1864 (3.65%)*	18/857 (2.10%)*	86/2721 (3.16%)

*p = 0.043, Chi-square test, Blacks vs Caucasians

Table 2 Distribution of Paraprotein Types

	Black	Caucasian	Total
IgG kappa/IgG lambda	43/19	7/3	50/22
IgA kappa/IgA lambda	4/5	1/0	5/5
IgM kappa/IgM lambda	3/2	7/1	10/3
Total kappa/lambda	50/26	15/4	65/30

DISCUSSION

Similar to the increased incidence of multiple myeloma in Black individuals, this study has demonstrated a 1.7-fold increase in the frequency of benign paraproteinemia in Blacks as compared to Caucasians. The paraproteinemia was also noted at an earlier age in the Black patients, similar to the age distribution of multiple myeloma in Black patients as compared to Caucasian patients (Blattner, 1980).

The distribution of paraprotein types also differed between the two groups. There was a marked predominance of IgG and IgA, the paraproteins associated with myeloma, with only 5 of the 68 Black patients (7%) having IgM paraproteins. In contrast, 8 of 18 of the Caucasian patients (44%) had IgM paraproteins.

Since the subjects of this study were hospitalized patients there is a concern that the increased prevalence of paraproteinemia we noted may have reflected factors related to acute or chronic illness. However, the frequency of benign paraproteinemia in our Caucasian patients, 2.1%, was only slightly higher than that previously described in predominantly white populations of similar age (Kyle, 1982). For example Kyle et al (1972) found a prevalence of 1.25% of paraproteinemia among 1200 residents over the age of 50 of a small Minnesota community.

Our results suggest that the factors playing a role in the increased susceptibility of Black individuals to develop multiple myeloma may also result in an increased propensity to form plasma cell clones of limited growth potential which result in the syndrome of benign paraproteinemia.

REFERENCES

Blattner WA (1980) Epidemiology of multiple myeloma and related plasma cell disorders: an analytic review. In: Potter M (ed) Progress in Myeloma. Elsevier, North Holland, New York, p 1

Kyle RA, Finkelstein S, Elveback LE, Kurland LT (1972) Incidence of monoclonal proteins in a Minnesota community with a cluster of multiple myeloma. Blood 40: 719-724

Kyle RA (1982) Monoclonal gammopathy of undetermined significance (MGUS): A review. Clin in Hematol 11:123-149

Schechter GP, Shoff N, Chan C, Hawley HP (1986) The frequency of asymptomatic mono- and biclonal gammopathy in hospitalized black and caucasian veterans. Blood 68: 214a

Racial Differences in the Expression of Shared Idiotypes by Paraproteins from Patients with Monoclonal Gammopathies

J.R. Berenson[1], A.K. Lichtenstein[1], J. Cao[1], S. Hart[2], D. Palomares[2], and R.A. Miller[2]

Department of Medicine[1], Wadsworth and Jonsson Cancer Centers, UCLA School of Medicine and VA West Los Angeles, Los Angeles, CA, and IDEC Pharmaceuticals Corporation[2], Mountain View, CA.

ABSTRACT

Twenty-nine murine monoclonal antibodies have been produced which react with shared idiotypes expressed by B-cell lymphomas and leukemias. We tested this panel of antibodies for reactivity with the paraproteins from 37 patients with multiple myeloma and 13 patients with monoclonal gammopathy of undetermined significance (MGUS). Fourteen of 50 paraproteins reacted with at least one antibody in this panel of anti-idiotypic antibodies. Seven different anti-idiotypes demonstrated reactivity with the paraproteins. A similar frequency of reactivity was found for both myeloma and MGUS proteins. One antibody, S30-47, reacted with eight (16%) of the paraproteins from patients with these monoclonal gammopathies; whereas, this anti-idiotype only bound to 3% of non-Hodgkin's B-cell lymphomas and no cases of chronic lymphocytic leukemia. This antibody demonstrated reactivity with paraproteins obtained from nearly one-third of black patients but none of the white patients' paraproteins showed reactivity with this anti-idiotype. In each of eleven patients tested, plasma cells isolated from bone marrow were shown to be reactive with the same anti-idiotype we found to react with the paraprotein. Anti-shared idiotype antibodies may provide useful reagents for studies of patients with monoclonal gammopathies.

INTRODUCTION

Immunoglobulin (Ig) molecules are composed of heavy and light chains, which possess highly specific variable regions at their amino termini. Regions of heavy and light chains combine to form the unique antigen-recognition structure of the Ig protein. These variable regions contain determinants which can themselves be recognized as antigens or idiotypes (Ids). Antibodies produced against these determinants are known as anti-Ids (Kunkel et al. 1970).

B cell malignancies are composed of clonal proliferations of cells synthesizing an antibody molecule with unique variable regions in the heavy and light chain (V_H and V_L). These cells express idiotypic determinants which are recognized by anti-Id antibodies (Stevenson and Stevenson 1975) and can serve as targets for diagnosis, treatment, and studies of these malignancies (Stevenson et al. 1977; Miller et al. 1982; Meeker et al. 1985; Brown et al. 1989). Anti-Ids have been used successfully for treatment of B cell malignancies (Miller et al. 1982; Meeker et al. 1985; Brown et al. 1989; Krolick et al. 1982; Perek et al. 1983). Studies employing anti-Id antibodies for human B cell lymphomas have been hindered by the requirement for producing a customized antibody for each patient's tumor. Recently, a panel of anti-Ids was produced which reacted with shared Ids expressed by the tumors of multiple patients with low-grade lymphomas (Miller et al 1989). One-third of B-cell lymphomas cases tested were shown to react with anti-Ids which were generated against Ids isolated from the tumors of other patients.

In this report, we examined paraproteins from patients with multiple myeloma and monoclonal gammopathy of undetermined significance (MGUS) for reactivity with this panel of anti-Id antibodies. These studies were undertaken to determine if relationships exist between the Ids expressed by B-cell lymphomas and another B cell lineage tumor, multiple myeloma, and its related disorder MGUS. Because there are distinct racial differences in the incidence of multiple myeloma in blacks and whites (McPhedran et al. 1972; Blattner 1980), we also determined whether the expression of these anti-shared idiotypes in paraproteins differed in black and white patients with these diseases.

METHODS

Patients

Thirty-seven patients with multiple myeloma were studied who fulfilled the diagnostic criteria of the Chronic Leukemia-Myeloma Task Force (Committee of the Chronic Leukemia-Myeloma Task Force 1973). Thirteen patients with MGUS also were evaluated and have been followed for three to nine years without increases in their serum paraprotein levels (Kyle 1978). This study was approved by Human Subject Protection Committees at both UCLA and the VAMC West Los Angeles.

Preparation of Anti-Idiotypic Antibodies

Id proteins were obtained from specimens of B-cell lymphomas according to previously described procedures using a heterohybridoma fusion technique (Carrol et al. 1986). Purified Id obtained from B cell tumors was used to immunize either mice or rats as previously described (Thielemans et al. 1984). Spleen cells were fused with the nonsecreting mouse myeloma line SP2/0 Ag 14, and hybridoma supernatants were screened for anti-Id reactivity (Miller et al. 1989). Anti-Ids were selected based on reactivity with the patient's Id but not with a panel of other antibodies, some of which were isotype matched. Anti-Ids reactive with shared Ids were found by using normal human serum to inhibit binding of anti-Id to the Id as previously described (Miller et al. 1989). Anti-Ids which reacted with low levels of serum Ig were tested for reactivity with lymphoma biopsy specimens. Antibodies reactive with tumors from more than one patient detected shared idiotypes. Twenty-nine out of a total of 43 anti-Ids identified using these techniques were used in the studies reported here. We have previously reported on the frequency of anti-shared Id reactivity with B cell lymphomas and leukemias (Miller et al. 1989). These results have now been extended to evaluate 306 cases of B cell lymphoma and 61 cases of chronic lymphocytic leukemia (CLL). The frequency of anti-shared Id reactivity with paraproteins is compared to the results obtained with B cell lymphomas and leukemias using the panel of 29 anti-Ids.

Detection of Shared Idiotypes Expressed by Paraproteins from Patients with Myeloma and MGUS

Sera from patients or normal donors were diluted 1:1000 and further serially diluted in a blocking solution containing 5% Carnation instant milk in phosphate buffered saline. This large dilution was performed to reduce the concentration of normal polyclonal Ig in the serum samples. Diluted sera from normal donors were tested in parallel with patients in these assays and showed no reactivity with any of the anti-shared Id antibodies. The diluted serum was incubated in the wells of microtiter plates coated with either goat $F(ab')_2$ anti-human Ig kappa light chain reagents (Tago, Burlingame, CA) for kappa paraproteins or anti-human Ig lambda light chains (Tago) for lambda paraproteins . The wells were washed, and the murine monoclonal anti-shared Ids were added. After incubation and washing, horseradish peroxidase conjugated goat anti-mouse IgG (Tago) was added to the wells. Bound antibody was detected by washing and adding 2,2'-AZINO-bis(3-ethylbenzthiazoline-6-sulfonic acid) (ABTS) substrate. Optical density (OD) was measured using a microtiter plate reader. A paraprotein was considered positive for reactivity with an anti-shared Id if the OD at a dilution of 1:1000 dilution was greater than three times that seen with normal serum. Non-reactive anti-shared Ids served as additional negative controls.

Shared Idiotype Expression by Bone Marrow Plasma Cells

Mononuclear cells were isolated from the bone marrow aspirates of nine patients by centrifugation through Histopaque 1077 (Pharmacia, Piscataway, NJ). Mononuclear cells were deposited on slides using a cytocentrifuge. The specimens were incubated with either the anti-shared Id which had been shown to react with the patient's paraprotein or other anti-Ids which were non-reactive with the paraprotein.. After washing, the slides were incubated with a biotinylated rabbit anti-mouse Ig reagent (Tago). After additional washing, an alkaline phosphatase conjugated avidin (Tago) was added. The substrate naphthol AS-MX phosphate mixed with Fast Red TR salt was added for color development. The slide was counterstained with hematoxylin #3 and examined using a light microscope.

RESULTS

Detection of Shared Idiotypes in Myeloma and MGUS Sera

Paraproteins from 14out of 50 patients reacted with anti-shared Id antibodies previously generated against B cell lymphomas. The reactive paraproteins contained a variety of light and heavy chain types (Table 1).

Table 1. Frequency of Reactivity of Paraproteins with Anti-Shared Idiotype Antibodies

Ig Class and Light Chain		Paraproteins with Shared Idiotypes Total # Tested
IgG kappa		5/26
IgG lambda		5/14
IgG kappa and lambda		1/1
IgA kappa		1/3
IgA lambda		1/5
IgM kappa		1/1
Subtotals:	Myeloma	10/37
	MGUS[a]	4/13
Totals:		14/50

[a]MGUS, monoclonal gammopathy of undetermined significance

IgG kappa proteins from five of 26 patients demonstrated reactivity. Five of 14 patients with IgG lambda paraproteins showed reactivity with the antibody panel. In one patient with a biphenotypic paraprotein, both the IgG kappa and IgG lambda paraproteins showed reactivity with the same anti-Id (Tables 1 and 2).

Table 2. Anti-Shared Idiotypes Reactive With Paraproteins

MAB[a]	# of Patients Reactive	Isotype
S30-47	8 (6 MM[b] and 2 MGUS[c])	1 IgG1 lambda 1 IgG3 lambda 1 IgG3 kappa 1 IgG4 kappa 3 IgG* kappa 1 IgG* lambda&kappa
J18-76	2 (2 MM)	1 IgG1 lambda 1 IgA lambda
H101-2	1 (1 MM)	IgA kappa
H-55-4	1 (1 MM)	IgG1 lambda
C31-145	1 (1 MGUS)	IgM kappa
S26-16	1 (1 MGUS)	IgG1 lambda[@]
W57-30	1 (1 MGUS)	IgG1 lambda[@]

[a]MAB, murine monoclonal anti-shared idiotype antibody; [b]MM, multiple myeloma; [c]MGUS, monoclonal gammopathy of undetermined significance; [@]both S26-26 and W57-30 reacted with the same IgG1 lambda MGUS paraprotein; *IgG isotype not determined

One patient each with IgA kappa, IgA lambda, and IgM kappa paraproteins reacted with anti-shared Id antibodies. Overall, nearly one-third (10/37) of myeloma paraproteins reacted with the anti-shared Ids. No differences were found in the age of patients, sex, stage, or response to therapy between patients with or without reactivity to anti-shared idiotypes. A similar fraction (4/13) of paraproteins from patients with MGUS showed reactivity.

Seven of the panel of 29 monoclonal anti-Ids reacted with these M-proteins (Table 2). One antibody, S30-47, reacted with paraproteins from six cases of myeloma including the patient with biphenotypic disease and two patients with MGUS. These patients had paraproteins which contained a variety of IgG heavy chain isotypes and either kappa or lambda light chains. Two myeloma patients' paraproteins reacted with the J18-76 antibody. Interestingly, proteins from two of the three MGUS patients demonstrated reactivity with anti-Ids which did not react with any of the myeloma M-proteins.

We compared the frequencies of anti-Id reactivity with paraproteins compared to their reactivity with the Ids expressed by B-cell lymphoma and CLL (Table 3). The overall reactivity of the anti-shared Ids with these three malignancies (27-39%) did not differ significantly. However, particular antibodies reacted with each of the types of B cell tumors at different frequencies. Most notable was S30-47 which reacted with 16% of myeloma but only 3% and 0% of lymphoma and CLL, respectively. Many anti-Ids which were reactive with the lymphoma and/or CLL samples did not show reactivity with any myeloma paraprotein. Thus, a different pattern of reactivity emerged with our myelomas than the other two B cell tumors.

Table 3. Reactivity of Anti-Shared Idiotypes with Different B Cell Malignancies

MAB[b]	MM[b]	NHL[c]	CLL[d]
S30-47	16%	3%	0%
J18-76	5	ND	ND
H55-4	3	0.4	3
H101-2	3	0	0
S37-48	0	4	6
C33-13	0	2	5
C45-23	0	2	4
C52-22	0	3	0
Others[e]	0	20	21
Totals:	27	34	39

[a]MAB, anti-shared idiotype antibody; [b]MM, 32 multiple myelomas; [c]NHL, 306 non-Hodgkin's lymphomas; [d]CLL, 61 chronic lymphocytic leukemias; [e]Others' includes 21 other anti-Ids which reacted with lymphomas and 9 other anti-Ids which reacted with CLL samples

Because marked differences in the incidence of myeloma exist between blacks and whites (McPhedran et al. 1972; Blattner 1980), we determined whether the reactivity of these anti-shared idiotypes was different in paraproteins from black and white patients (Table 4).

Table 4. Racial Differences in Reactivity of Anti-Shared Idiotypes

MAB[a]	Black	White
S30-47	8/26	0/21
H55-4	1/26	0/21
J18-76	1/26	1/21
C31-145	0/26	1/21
H101-2	0/26	1/21*
S26-16	0/26	1/21
W57-30	0/26	1/21*
Totals:	10/26	4/21

[a]MAB, anti-shared idiotype antibody; * one patient reacted with two antiidiotypes

Interestingly, S30-47 reacted with nearly one-third (8/26) of the paraproteins obtained from black patients but did not show reactivity with any of the paraproteins produced by 21 white patients. In order to show that this anti-idiotype was not reactive with normal black serum, it was tested on diluted (1:1000) serum from 19 control black patients without paraproteins. None of these control patients' serum reacted with S30-47. Overall reactivity was higher in black (10/26) than white patients (4/21) but these differences were due to the marked difference in reactivity with S30-47 between these two racial groups.

Demonstration of Shared Idiotype Expression by the Bone Marrow Plasma Cells

In each of eleven cases studied, the bone marrow plasma cells showed marked reactivity with the same anti-Id that was found to be reactive with the patient's paraprotein. Plasma cells and approximately 80% of the lymphoid cells in these patients' marrow specimens were reactivewith the anti-Ids. Figure 1 shows the results of immunocytochemical staining using the H55-4 anti-Id on bone marrow cells from a patient with IgG1 lambda myeloma. The patient's plasma cells and lymphocytes show staining with this antibody which also reacted with the patient's paraprotein.

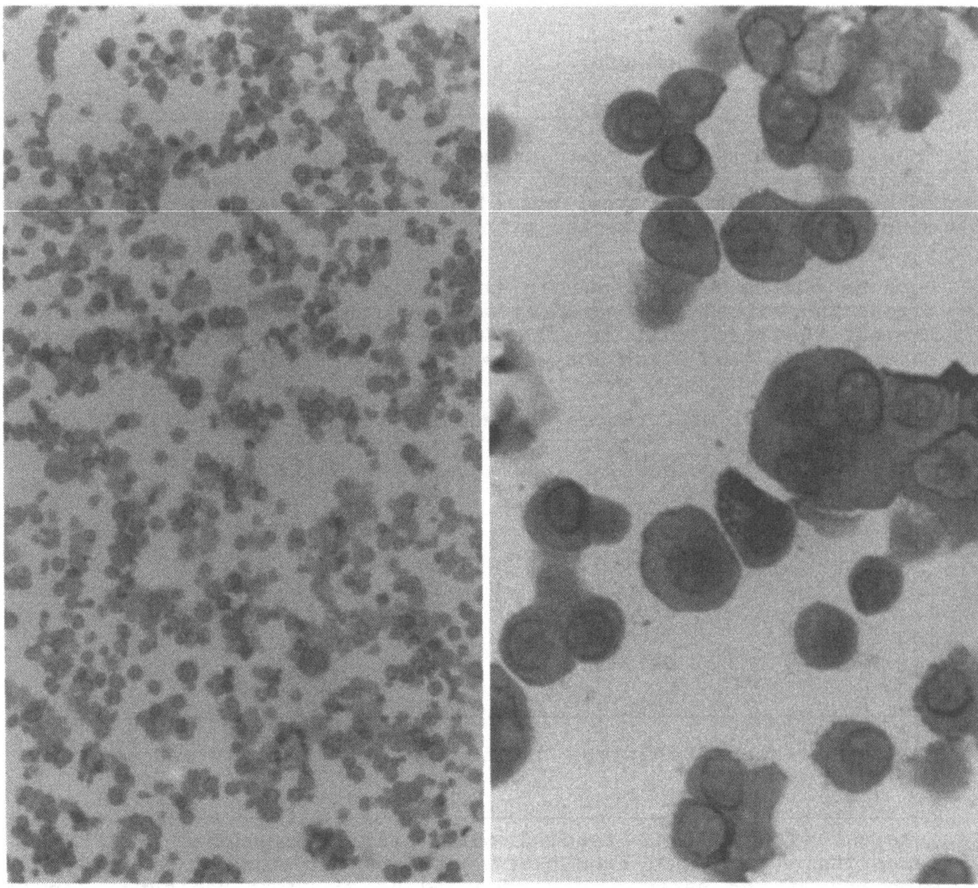

Fig. 1. Immunocytochemical staining of a cytocentrifuge specimen from a bone marrow of a patient with IgG1 kappa myeloma. The cells were stained with H55-4. Cells are shown both at low (100X) magnification and higher (400X) magnification. Many cells react with the anti-idiotype, and under higher magnification these reactive cells are shown to be plasma and lymphoid cells.

Bone marrow from two patients with MGUS were tested for reactivity with anti-Ids that reacted with their paraprotein. In these two cases, greater than 90% of the plasma cells reacted with the anti-Id.

DISCUSSION

Shared Ids have been described in non-malignant B cell disorders including: systemic lupus erythematosus (SLE), rheumatoid arthritis, mixed cryoglobulinemia, and IgA nephropathy (Goni et al. 1985; Kunkel et al. 1973; Isenberg et al. 1984; Gonzalez-Cabrero et al. 1987; Mageed et al. 1988), as well as in a number of B cell malignancies (Miller et al. 1989; Kipps 1988; Kipps et al. 1988a; Kipps et al. 1989; Davidson et al. 1987). Davidson and co-workers showed that an anti-Id which recognized a determinant on kappa-chains of anti-DNA antibodies in SLE patients also reacted with over 10% of myelomas (Davidson et al. 1987). Recently, Miller et al. demonstrated that a high proportion of B-cell lymphomas express shared Ids using a panel of anti-Ids generated against follicular lymphomas (Miller et al. 1989). Using these anti-shared idiotype antibodies, we have demonstrated that one-third of myeloma and MGUS paraproteins react with anti-Id antibodies that were generated against low-grade follicular B-cell lymphomas.

Two antibodies known as 17.109 and G6 were generated against rheumatoid factors and react with the cells of up to 20% of patients with CLL (Kipps 1988; Kipps et al. 1988a; Kipps et al. 1989). The frequent occurrence of Ids reacting with the two anti-Id antibodies has been shown to be the result of the expression of a few Ig germline V genes (Kipps 1988; Kipps et al. 1988a). The G6 and 17.109 antibodies show reactivity much less frequently with B-cell lymphomas (Kipps 1988; Kipps et al. 1988a). In previous studies, B-cell lymphomas were shown to express shared Ids in about one-third of cases (Miller et al. 1989). However, the frequency of reactivity with particular anti-Ids in lymphoma is lower than that observed in CLL (Miller et al. 1989; Kipps et al. 1989). In our current study of monoclonal gammopathies, we find that one anti-Id, S30-47, reacts with a high proportion (17%) of paraproteins. It is likely that this anti-Id is directed against a Ig heavy chain determinant because it reacts with both the IgG kappa and IgG lambda paraproteins in our patient with biphenotypic myeloma, The frequency of reactivity of S30-47 with B-cell lymphomas (3.6%) was less than that sees with the monoclonal gammopathies, it was one of the most frequently reactive anti-Ids with B-cell lymphomas (Miller et al. 1989). Overall, different antibody reactivity was seen with myeloma, CLL, and lymphomas. These results suggest that these B cell lineage malignancies evolve from different B cell subsets or are potentially driven by different antigenic stimuli. In support of this, it is known that CLL and B-cell lymphoma use different V_H genes preferentially (Kipps 1988; Kipps et al. 1988a; Humphries et al. 1988). In addition, B-cell lymphomas have an active Ig somatic mutational process (Cleary et al. 1986); whereas CLL does not exhibit hypermutation (Kipps 1988; Kipps et al. 1988b; Meeker et al. 1988). In murine plasmacytomas, frequent somatic mutation occurs (Kim et al. 1981). In order to determine which V genes are utilized and the rate of somatic mutation, it will be necessary to sequence the V genes expressed by the plasma cells in patients with myeloma.

The incidence of multiple myeloma in blacks is twice that observed in white patients (McPhedran et al. 1972; Blattner 1980), and, in fact, it represents the most common lymphoreticular malignancy in blacks (Blattner 1980). The reason for these apparent racial differences have been theorized to result from either environmental chemical or antigenic exposures and/or genetic predisposition. In our studies, we show marked differences in the reactivity of paraproteins with this panel of anti-shared idiotypes. Specifically, one anti-idiotype, S30-47, reacts with nearly one-third of paraproteins from black patients but does not react with the proteins from white patients. Other anti-shared idiotypes also showed racial differences. A larger series of patients will be necessary to show the significance of these latter differences in racial idiotypic reactivity. However, these preliminary studies suggest differences in V gene usage in the paraproteins produced by these two racial groups. Whether these variations reflect racial differences in V gene usage during normal B cell function or reflect differences in exposure to specific environmental antigens is unknown. However, the amount of idiotype reactive with S30-47 in sera obtained from control patients without monoclonal gammopathies is similar in blacks and whites. This would imply that normal expression of V genes leading to production of immunoglobulins with S30-47 reactivity is similar in blacks and whites.

There is some evidence suggesting that myeloma may originate from an earlier cell in B cell differentiation than the plasma cell (Kubagawa et al. 1979). The S30-47 reacted with both the IgG kappa and IgG lambda paraprotein components in a patient with biphenotypic myeloma. This suggests that in this patient the tumor is clonal and that the original malignant event occurred in a cell that had not yet undergone light chain rearrangement. Alternatively, a malignant cell may have sustained a mutation which rendered the kappa chain gene nonproductive leading to the productive rearrangement of the lambda chain gene.

The frequency of shared Id expression in monoclonal gammopathies of both the malignant form, multiple myeloma, and the relatively benign state, MGUS, appeared to be similar. In some cases, the same anti-Id reacted with both myeloma and MGUS. Two monoclonal anti-Ids reacted only with MGUS patients. It will require a larger series of patients in order to determine if the shared Ids detected by these two anti-Ids are restricted to MGUS paraproteins. The existence of some Ids which are shared by both myelomas and B-cell lymphomas suggests that some of these tumors may utilize the same V genes. In CLL which is a malignancy of CD5 positive B-cells, limited V gene usage is thought to represent the restricted repertoire of CD5 positive cells which are utilized during early B-cell ontogeny. In support of this, it is known that CD5 positive cells constitute the predominant B-cell population in human fetal liver and spleen (Bofill et al. 1985; Antin et al. 1986). Some malignant cells in multiple myeloma also have been shown to express CD5 (Duperray et al. 1989).

We found that bone marrow plasma cells isolated from patients reacted with the same anti-Id that bound to their paraproteins. In preliminary studies, we have seen similar reactivity with a subpopulation of peripheral blood lymphocytes from patients with myeloma (unpublished observations). These anti-Ids provide an opportunity to identify and isolate the malignant cells from the blood as well as the marrow. The identification of Id-bearing plasma cells in the normal appearing marrow of MGUS patients suggests that these cells are responsible for production of the paraprotein in this disorder.

In this study, the anti-shared Ids which bind to the myeloma and MGUS paraproteins were prepared against follicular lymphomas. By producing antibodies against myeloma or MGUS paraproteins directly, one may be able to identify anti-Ids with more frequent reactivity with paraproteins. It is possible that the B cell tumors expressing specific shared Ids represent distinct subsets of these malignancies with distinct pathophysiologies, clinical characteristics and prognoses. In support of this, marked racial differences were found in the reactivity of these anti-Ids with paraproteins obtained from black and white patients.

Anti-shared Id antibodies should facilitate studies of the biology of B cell malignancies including multiple myeloma. These antibodies may be used to investigate relationships between myeloma and MGUS. Using the techniques described in this report, these reagents also may find a valuable role in diagnosis and/or monitoring of monoclonal gammopathies.

REFERENCES

Antin JH, Emerson SG, Martin P, Gadol N, Ault KA (1975) Leu-1+ (CD5+) B cells. A major lymphoid subpopulation in human fetal spleen: Phenotypic and functional studies. J Immunol 136:505-510

Blattner WA (1980) Epidemiology of multiple myeloma and related plasma cell disorders: An analytic review. In: Potter M, ed. Progress in myeloma. New York:Elsevier/North Holland, Inc. p 1-65

Bofill M, Janossy G, Janossa M, Burford GD, Seymour GJ, Wernet P, Kelemen E (1985) Human B cell development: II. Subpopulations in the human fetus. J Immunol 134:1531-1538

Brown S, Miller RA, Horning SJ, Czerwinski D, Hart SM, McElderry R, Basham T, Warnke R, Merigan TC, Levy R (1989) Treatment of B-cell lymphomas with anti-idiotype antibodies alone and in combination with alpha interferon. Blood 73:651-661

Carrol WL, Thielemans K, Dilley J, Levy R (1986) Mouse x human heterohybridomas as fusion partners with human B cell tumors. J Immunol Methods 89:61-72

Cleary ML, Meeker TC, Levy S, Lee E, Trela M, Sklar J, Levy R (1986) Clustering of extensive somatic mutations in the variable region of an immunoglobulin heavy chain gene from a human B cell lymphoma. Cell 44:97-106

Committee of the Chronic Leukemia-Myeloma Task Force (1973) Proposed Guidelines for Protocol Studies. II. Plasma cell myeloma. Cancer Chemother Rep 4:145-158

Davidson A, Preud'homme JL, Solomon A, Chang MDY, Beede S, Diamond B (1987) Idiotypic analysis of myeloma proteins: anti-DNA activity of monoclonal immunoglobulins bearing an SLE idiotype is more common in IgG than IgM antibodies. J Immunol 138:1515-1518

Duperray C, Klein B, Durie BGM, Zhang X, Jourdan M, Poncelet P, Favier F, Vincent C, Brochier J, Lenoir G, Bataille R (1989) Phenotypic analysis of human myeloma cell lines. Blood 73:566-572

Goni F, Chen PP, Pons-Estel B, Carson DA, Frangione B (1985) Sequence similarities and cross-idiotypic specificity of L chains among human monoclonal IgM-K with anti-globulin activity. J Immunol 135: 4073-4079

Gonzalez-Cabrero, Egido J, Sancho J, Moldenhauer F (1987) Presence of shared idiotypes in serum and immune complexes in patients with IgA nephropathy. Clin Exp Immunol 68:694-702

Humphries CG, Shen A, Kuziel WA, Capra JD, Blattner FR, Tucker PW (1988) A new human immunoglobulin V_H family preferentially rearranged in immature B-cell tumours. Nature 331:446-449

Isenberg DA, Shoenfeld Y, Madaio MP, Rauch J, Reichlin M, Stollar BD, Schwartz RS (1984) Anti-DNA antibody idiotypes in systemic lupus erythematosus. Lancet ii:417-422

Kim S, Davis M, Sinn E, Patten P, Hood L (1981) Antibody diversity: somatic hypermutation of rearranged V_H genes. Cell 27:573-581

Kipps TJ (1988) Immunoglobulin V gene utilization in chronic lymphocytic leukemia and non-Hodgkin's B cell lymphomas. Nouv Rev Fr Hematol 30:293-298

Kipps TJ, Robbins BA, Kuster P, Carson DA (1988a) Autoantibody-associated cross-reactive idiotypes expressed at high frequency in chronic lymphocytic leukemia relative to B-cell lymphomas of follicular center cell origin. Blood 72:422-428

Kipps TJ, Tomhave E, Chen PP, Carson DA (1988b) Autoantibody-associated kappa light chain variable region gene expressed in chronic lymphocytic leukemia with little or no somatic mutation. J Exp Med 167:840-852

Kipps TJ, Tomhave E, Pratt LF, Duffy S, Chen PP, Carson D (1989) Developmentally restricted immunoglobulin heavy chain variable region gene expressed at high frequency in chronic lymphocytic leukemia. Proc Natl Acad Sci USA 86:5913-5917

Krolik KA, Uhr JW, Slavin S, Vitetta ES (1982) In vivo therapy of a murine B cell tumor (BCL1) using antibody-ricin A chain immunotoxins. J Exp Med 155:1797-1809

Kubagawa J, Vogler LB, Capra JD, Conrad ME, Lawton AR, Cooper M (1979) Study of the clonal origin of multiple myeloma. J Exp Med 150: 792-807

Kunkel HG, Mannik M, Williams RC (1963) Individual antigenic specificity of isolated antibodies. Science 140:1218-1219

Kunkel HG, Agnello V, Joslin FG, Winchester RJ, Capra JD (1973) Cross idiotypic specificity among monoclonal IgM proteins with anti-gammaglobulin activity. J Exp Med 137:331-342

Kyle RA (1978) Monoclonal gammopathy of undetermined significance: Natural history in 241 cases. Am J Med 64:814-826

Mageed RA, Carson DA, Jefferis R (1988) Analysis of rheumatoid factor autoantibodies in patients with essential mixed cryoglobulinaenemia and rheumatoid arthritis. Scand J Rheumatol 75 (Suppl):172-178

McPhedran P, Heath CW Jr, Garcia J (1972) Multiple myeloma incidence in metropolitan Atlanta, Georgia: Racial and seasonal variations. Blood 39:866-873

Meeker TC, Lowder J, Maloney DG, Miller RA, Thielemans K, Warnke R, Levy R (1985) A clinical trial of anti-idiotype therapy for B cell malignancy. Blood 65:1349-1363

Meeker TC, Grimaldi JG, O'Rourke R, Loeb J, Juliusson G, Einhorn S (1988) Lack of detectable somatic hypermutation in the V region of an Ig H chain gene of a human chronic B lymphocytic leukemia. J Immunol 141:3994-3998

Miller RA, Maloney DG, Warnke R, and Levy R (1982) Treatment of B-cell lymphoma with monoclonal anti-idiotype antibody. N Eng J Med 306:517-522

Miller RA, Hart S, Samoszuk M, Coulter C, Brown S, Czerwinski D, Lelenberg J, Royston I, Levy R (1989) Shared idiotypes expressed by human B-cell lymphomas. N Eng J Med 321:851-857

Perek Y, Hurwitz E, Burowski D, Haimovich J (1983) Immunotherapy of a murine B cell tumor with antibodies and F $(ab')_2$ fragments against idiotypic determinants of its cell surface IgM. J Immunol 131: 1600-1603

Stevenson GT, Elliot EV, Stevenson FK (1977) Idiotypic determinants on the surface immunoglobulin of neoplastic lymphocytes: a therapeutic target. Fed Proc 36:2268-2271

Stevenson GT and Stevenson FK (1975) Antibody to a molecularly-defined antigen confined to a tumour cell surface. Nature 254:714-716

Thielemans K, Maloney DG, Meeker T, Fujimoto J, Doss C, Warnke RA, Bindl J, Gralow J, Miller RA, Levy R (1984) Strategies for production of monoclonal anti-idiotype antibodies against human B cell lymphomas. J Immunol 133:495-501

Etiologic Hypotheses

Is Chronic Antigenic Stimulation Etiologically Related to Multiple Myeloma ?

M.S. Linet

Analytic Studies Section, Biostatistics Branch, Epidemiology & Biostatistics Program, Division of Cancer Etiology, National Cancer Institute, Executive Plaza North Room 415B, Bethesda, MD 20892

INTRODUCTION

Beginning in 1958, case reports and surveys linked repeated immune stimulation from chronic infectious and inflammatory disorders (Isobe and Osserman, 1971; Schafer and Miller, 1979), connective tissue and autoimmune diseases (Abbatt and Lea, 1958; Talal and Bunim, 1964; Blackburn et al, 1968; Viadana and Bross, 1974; Isomaki et al, 1978) with an elevated risk of multiple myeloma, malignant lymphoma, leukemias, and other lymphoproliferative malignancies. Allergy-related conditions were associated with higher risk of myeloma and related lymphoproliferative neoplasms in a few reports (Penny and Hughes, 1970; McWhorter, 1988), but similar occurrence of Hodgkin's disease (Dworin et al, 1955) was observed among those with and without prior allergies (Dworin et al, 1955). The proliferative process involving myeloma and some other lymphoproliferative malignancy B cells was postulated to arise from repeated or continuous aberrant immunologic responses (Isobe and Osserman, 1971).

However, the suspect antigenic-stimulating conditions were often vaguely characterized (e.g., "rheumatic diseases" or "rheumatism") and consisted of disparate disorders. The lymphoproliferative malignancy outcomes also varied among the studies. Some investigations combined prevalent <u>and</u> incident cases, others lacked control groups, and most failed to consider latency or potential confounding factors. The notion of "chronic antigenic stimulation" was oversimplified, because an antigen that stimulates a suppressor T cell can produce a clinical state of immunodeficiency, for example. In addition, the chronic antigenic stimulation hypothesis postulated that the target cell was an end-stage, antibody-producing B cell, whereas cells at earlier stages of B cell development may be more important (Epstein et al, 1990). Nevertheless, the totality of findings was difficult to dismiss, particularly in light of animal models suggesting a relationship of myeloma and related lymphoproliferative malignancies with immune stimulation (Lee and Ihle, 1982; Potter, 1985). In the late 1970's several case-control studies were undertaken to test the hypothesis relating immune stimulation and myeloma.

IMMUNE-STIMULATING CONDITIONS AND MULTIPLE MYELOMA

Most of the epidemiologic studies assessed the clinical conditions linked with myeloma by Osserman and colleagues (Isobe and Osserman, 1971) including pyelonephritis, urinary tract infectious, prostatitis, bronchitis, tuberculosis, gallbladder disease, diverticulitis, skin infections, osteomyelitis, hepatitis, and peptic ulcer disease. Autoimmune disorders linked with myeloma were glomerulonephritis, thyroiditis, rheumatoid arthritis, and several other collagen vascular disorders. Allergy-related conditions and hyposensitization therapy were also associated with myeloma. The hypothesis evaluated was whether chronic infections, inflammatory, autoimmune, and allergy-related disorders were of higher prevalence in individuals who develop multiple myeloma compared with controls.

Gallagher et al (1983) in a population-based evaluation of 84 cases and controls in British Columbia found a positive association with prior allergies, allergy treatments, and myxedema. No link was noted for chronic infections, inflammatory conditions or autoimmune disorders. Among 76 hospital-based cases and controls in New Zealand, an elevated myeloma risk was seen among those with hayfever but not other allergies (Pearce et al, 1986). Cases were less likely to have received hyposensitization treatments than controls , but no association was found for history of asthma, eczema, drug allergies or rheumatoid arthritis. However, 153 hospital-based cases and controls at Duke-affiliated hospitals in Durham, North Carolina had significantly less prior immune-stimulation (an exposure variable defined prior to all analyses consisting of at least one of any of the conditions listed above from the paper by Isobe and Osserman) than controls (Cohen et al, 1987). The apparent protective effect persisted even when various subgroups of the hospital controls were excluded. No association with immune stimulation was noted among 100 hospital-based cases and controls in Baltimore (Linet et al, 1987).

Larger studies also failed to demonstrate consistent findings. Among 698 population-based cases and controls identified from four geographic areas in the U.S., small excesses were found among those with prior history of rheumatic fever, urinary tract infections, and shrapnel wounds (Koepsell et al, 1987). However, cases were less likely to have a history of prior allergies, hyposensitization treatments or hepatitis. Myeloma was inversely related to the number of diseases against which the subject was immunized but no association was found with the number of past viral or bacterial illnesses or hyposensitization injections. No associations were observed between allergy-related disorders, common childhood viral illnesses, immunization history and myeloma in a hospital-based study of 399 cases and controls in parts of the United Kingdom (Cuzick et al, 1988).

CONCLUSIONS

Case-control studies assessing past medical history of chronic infectious, inflammatory, connective tissue, autoimmune, and allergy-related disorders derived from interview of multiple myeloma cases and controls or their proxies have shown little support for the immune stimulation hypothesis of myeloma etiology, with the possible exception of a generally protective effect observed for prior allergy conditions. Inverse associations have also been found between allergy-related conditions and other hematolymphoproliferative neoplasms including chronic lymphocytic leukemia (Linet et al, 1986; Cartwright et al, 1987), non-Hodgkin's lymphoma (Tielsch et al, 1987), and acute myelocytic leukemia (Severson et al, 1989; McKinney et al, 1990). Most of the studies were too small to adequately evaluate the relationship of autoimmune and connective tissue disorders with multiple myeloma. Preliminary evidence suggests that immunologic subtypes of myeloma may be etiologically distinct (Schafer and Miller, 1979; Williams et al, 1989), with distinct risk factors observed for cases with light chain myeloma. It should be noted that interview-based approaches have many limitations. Use of additional data sources may be helpful, although interview-derived information may be more complete than medical record data for conditions such as allergy history (Linet et al, 1989). Many of the analyses combined medical conditions which may not be homogeneous in immunologic effects, and thus associations may have be masked.

Future research should include evaluation of immune stimulation with myeloma subtypes in the two larger studies (Koepsell et al, 1987; Cuzick et al, 1988). Another approach might involve follow-up of large "exposed" cohorts with the most promising of the antigen-stimulating conditions (such as rheumatoid arthritis), identified from populations served by high quality cancer registries and from which all persons with antigen-stimulating conditions and myeloma can be ascertained (see Hakulinen et al, 1985). The methods should include careful review of the clinical data of all persons with the suspect condition to identify a homogeneous "exposed" cohort, as well as expert immunopathologic review of myeloma cases arising in this cohort to determine subtypes for separate analysis. Understanding of pathogenesis and etiology might be substantially strengthened by serial immunologic function follow-up to include identification of the progression of abnormalities leading to onset of monoclonal gammopathy and/or myeloma. The most appropriate population to use for such a cohort investigation might therefore be a health maintenance organization. Finally, an important component of such a cohort study will be the types of standardized, relatively inexpensive and feasible immunologic function tests applicable to such a survey research study.

REFERENCES

Abbatt J, Lea AJ (1958) Leukaemogens. Lancet 2:880-883.

Blackburn EK, Callendar ST, Dacie JV, Doll R, Girdwood RH, Mollin DL, Saracci R, Stafford JL, Thompson RB, Varadi S, Wetherly-Mein G (1968) Possible association between pernicious anemia and leukemia: Prospective study of 1,625 patients with a note on the very high incidence of stomach cancer. Int J Cancer 3:163-170.

Cartwright RA, Bernard SM, Bird CC, Darwin CM, O'Brien C, Richards IDG, Roberts B, McKinney PA (1987) Chronic lymphocytic leukemia: case-control epidemiological study in Yorkshire. Br J Cancer 56:79-82.

Cohen HJ, Bernstein RJ, Grufferman S (1987) Role of immune stimulation in the etiology of multiple myeloma: A case control study. Am J Hematol 24:119-126.

Cuzick J, De Stavola B (1988) Multiple myeloma-A case-control study. Br J Cancer 57:516-520.

Dworin M, Diamond HD, Craver LF (1955) Hodgkin's disease and allergy. Cancer 8:128-131.

Epstein J Xiao H, He X-Y (1990) Markers of multiple hematopoietic-cell lineages in multiple myeloma. N Engl J Med 322:664-668.

Gallagher RP, Spinelli JJ, Elwood JM, Skippen DH (1983) Allergies and agricultural exposure as risk factors for multiple myeloma. Br J Cancer 48:853-857.

Hakulinen T, Isomaki H, Knekt P (1985) Rheumatoid arthritis and cancer studies based on linking nationwide registries in Finland. Am J Med 78(Suppl 1A):29-32.

Isobe T, Osserman EF (1971) Pathologic conditions associated with plasma cell dyscrasias: A study of 806 cases. Ann NY Acad Sci 190:507-518.

Isomaki HA, Hakulinen T, Jousenlahti U (1978) Excess risk of lymphomas, leukemia and myeloma in patients with rheumatoid arthritis. J Chronic Dis 31:691-696.

Koepsell TD, Daling JR, Weiss NS, Taylor JW, Olshan AF, Lyon JL, Swanson GM, Child M (1987) Antigenic stimulation and the occurrence of multiple myeloma. Am J Epidemiol 126:1051-1062.

Lee JC, Ihle JN (1982) Chronic immune stimulation is required for Moloney leukaemia virus-induced lymphomas. Nature 289:407-409.

Linet MS, Harlow SD, McLaughlin JK (1987) A case-control study of multiple myeloma in whites: Chronic antigenic stimulation, occupation, and drug use. Cancer Res 47:2978-2981.

Linet MS, Harlow SD, McLaughlin JK, McCaffrey LD (1989) A comparison of interview data and medical records for previous medical conditions and surgery. J Clin Epidemiol 42:1207-1213.
Linet MS, McCaffrey LD, Humphrey RL, Brookmeyer R, Van Natta ML, Tielsch JM, Bias WB, Markowitz JA, Kravitz SC, Szklo M (1986) Chronic lymphocytic leukemia and acquired disorders affecting the immune system: A case-control study. JNCI 77:371-378.
McKinney PA, Alexander FE, Roberts BE, O'Brien C, Bird CC, Cartwright RA (1990) Yorkshire case control study of leukemias and lymphomas: Parallel multivariate analysis of seven disease categories. Leuk Lymph (in press)
McWhorter WP (1988) Allergy and risk of cancer. A prospective study using NHANES-I followup data. Cancer 62:451-455.
Pearce NE, Smith AH, Howard JK, Sheppard RA, Giles HJ, Teague CA (1986) Case-control study of multiple myeloma and farming. Br J Cancer 54:493-500.
Penny R, Hughes S (1970) Repeated stimulation of the reticuloendothelial system and the development of plasma-cell dyscrasias. Lancet 1:77.
Potter M (1985) Concepts of pathogenesis and experimental models of immunoglobulin-secreting tumors in animals. In: Wiernik PH, Canellos GP, Kyle RA, Schiffer CA (eds) Neoplastic diseases of the blood. Churchchill Livingstone, New York, p 393.
Schafer AI, Miller JB (1979) Association of IgA multiple myeloma with pre-existing disease. Br J Haematol 41:19-24.
Severson RK, Davis S, Thomas DB, Stevens RG, Heuser L, Sever LE (1989) Acute myelocytic leukemia and prior allergies. J Clin Epidemiol 42:995-1001.
Talal N, Bunim JJ (1964) The development of malignant lymphoma in the course of Sjogren's syndrome. Am J Med 36:529-540.
Tielsch JM, Linet MS, Szklo M (1987) Acquired disorders affecting the immune system and non-Hodgkin's lymphoma. Prev Med 16:96-106.
Viadana I, Bross ID (1974) Use of the medical history to predict the future occurrence of leukemias in adults. Prev Med 3:165-170.
Williams AR, Weiss NS, Koepsell TD, Lyon JL, Swanson GM (1989) Infectious and noninfectious exposures in the etiology of light chain myeloma: A case-control study. Cancer Res 49:4038-4041.

The Etiology of Multiple Myeloma: A Role for Viruses ?

N. Mueller

Department of Epidemiology, Harvard School of Public Health, 677 Huntington Avenue, Boston, MA 02115, USA

INTRODUCTION

Multiple myeloma (MM) is a malignancy which presents a complex picture of immune dysfunction. There is abnormal production of monoclonal antibody coupled with a diminished capacity to produce antibody in general. Impairment in cellular immunity is also apparent (Jacobson and Zolla-Pazner 1986). The abnormal plasma cells have low proliferative activity *in vitro*, requiring the presence of macrophages or IL-6 for continuing growth (Barlogie, this meeting). There is active suppression of antibody synthesis which is mediated by a immunoregulatory B cell (MacKenzie et al. 1987). Increased lymphotoxin production appears to be responsible for the bone destruction and hypercalcemia seen in patients (Garrett et al. 1987). Cytogenic abnormalities are common, typically involving chromosomes and sites related to immune regulatory genes, yet no consistent abnormality nor oncogene is present (MacKenzie and Lewis 1985, Selvanayagam et al. 1988).

The picture which emerges is of a disease process in which sustained antigenic stimulation of the antibody-producing arm of the immune system has induced an alteration in lymphokine production, leading to the uncontrolled production of monoclonal plasma cells and the accompanying immune dysfunction. The purpose of this paper is to address the question of whether a viral infection may play a role in this process.

VIRAL ONCOGENESIS

Accumulating epidemiologic and virologic evidence demonstrates that in a variety of malignancies - primarily those of the hemopoietic system - viruses play an etiologic role (Mueller et al. 1990). The viruses involved share in common the ability to establish latency. The mechanisms involved appear to cluster in two groups. The first involves malignancies in which there is always monoclonal integration of viral genome suggesting a mutational or initiating role. An example of this is the role of the human T-cell leukemia virus-I in adult T-cell leukemia/lymphoma (Yoshida, et al. 1984).

A less direct role can be seen in those malignancies where the associated viral genome is not usually integrated in the malignant cells but rather, there is evidence of chronic viral expression preceding disease occurrence. In this case, the virus appears to have played a mitogenic or promotional role in oncogenesis. An example of this would be the role of hepatitis B virus in chronic carriers who develop primary hepatocellular carcinoma.

The Epstein-Barr Virus in Non-Hodgkin's Lymphoma

An example in which chronically reactivated virus prior to the diagnosis of malignancy has been well documented involves the Epstein-Barr virus (EBV) and the occurrence of non-Hodgkin's lymphoma (NHL). This has been observed in two populations. The first includes organ transplant patients following therapeutic immunosuppression. Such patients have a greatly increased risk of NHL, often occurring within a few months of transplantation. Ho et al. (1985) have described 13 such patients who developed NHL or lymphoproliferative lesions following organ transplantation. Serum samples were collected before or at the time of transplantation and at least monthly for up to a year following. Based on antibody assays on the serial specimens, it was found that 6 of these patients experienced primary EBV infection and the rest, reactivated latent infection following their transplant. Prior to malignancy these patients characteristically had elevated antibody titers against the viral capsid antigen (VCA) of EBV, including IgG, IgM and IgA. Antibodies against the early antigen (EA) - indicative of viral replication - were also elevated. However, antibodies against the nuclear antigen (EBNA) were low or absent. Nine of 11 of these tumors contained EBV genome detected by DNA-DNA hybridization.

The progression of events in these therapeutically immunosuppressed patients is that with loss of cellular immunity-mediated control of EBV infection, there are repeated cycles of replication as evidenced by this serologic profile. A polyclonal proliferation of EBV-infected B cells occurs which in some persons, with the continuing mitogenic stimulation by repeated viral replication, becomes a monoclonal proliferation. Withdrawal or reduction of immunosuppression can result in a reversion of the malignancy (List et al. 1987). Hoover (personal communication) has pointed out that these characteristics of a late-acting, reversible mitogenic effect are indicative of a promotional role. Thus, in this situation, the antibody profile to the EBV provides epidemiologic evidence of promotion.

Recently, we evaluated the EBV antibody levels in blood specimens obtained from individuals who subsequently developed NHL. This study was part of a large collaborative undertaking combining the resources of four population-based serum collections with specimens from 238,000 individuals, for whom subsequent cancer diagnoses could be identified.[1] In these populations, there were 104 persons for whom specimens had been collected on average 63 months (range 6-168 months) prior to the diagnosis of NHL. For comparison, specimens from 259 matched controls were also analyzed. The EBV antibody profile for these "spontaneous" malignancies was quite similar to that seen for organ transplant patients who develop NHL. This suggests that chronic EBV expression plays either a direct, promotional role in the etiology of some lymphomas, or at least, is a strong indicator of immune dysregulation. (Mueller et al. 1990).

A VIRAL ETIOLOGY OF MULTIPLE MYELOMA

The question before us then is whether similar mechanisms are evident for MM. To my knowledge, there are no published reports of evidence of integrated viral genome in MM cells, including the EBV (Epstein et al. 1990), suggestive of an initiative role. A more attractive hypothesis is that a chronically reactive B-cell-tropic virus plays a promotional role, since the immunologic picture of MM is one involving chronic antigenic pressure on B-cells. The EBV is a candidate virus as it immortalizes B-cells. In the larger study described above, we also evaluated patients who developed MM following the collection of

[1]The co-principal investigators include: A. Evans, N.L. Harris, G.W. Comstock, E. Jellum, K. Magnus, N. Orentreich, B.F. Polk, and J. Vogelman. The collections and study design are described in Mueller, et al. 1989. A. Mohar was responsible for analysis of NHL data.

blood specimens. Details of this study will be published elsewhere.[2] In brief, 24 individuals were identified from whom blood specimens had been obtained a mean of 69 months (range 12-168) prior to a diagnosis of MM. Specimens from 66 matched controls were analyzed for comparison. Unlike the pre-disease EBV antibody profile seen for NHL patients, antibody titers against the VCA and EA were substantially reduced among the MM patients. Those against EBNA were somewhat reduced. This pre-diagnosis profile is not consistent with a promotional role for EBV in the etiology of MM.

CONCLUSIONS

Chronic antigenic stimulation from reactivated latent viral infections may play a promotional role in the induction of MM. No known virus has been linked to the disease. Characteristics of a candidate virus include that it is a highly prevalent lymphotropic infection (especially in the Black community), and has the ability to remain as a persistent infection with periodic reactivation. The existence of the Aleutian mink virus model argues that a similar unknown human retrovirus may also exist.

Future studies should focus on the identification of new viruses from tissue specimens (bone marrow, spleen and perhaps lymph nodes) of patients. The new techniques to detect retroviruses which have emerged from the AIDS epidemic will be of value in this search. In addition, prospective follow-up of monoclonal gammopathy patients should be carried out for evaluation of antibody profiles of candidate viruses and for confirmation of our EBV-antibody findings. In sum, whether a virus plays a role in the etiology of MM is presently unknown, but by combining epidemiologic and molecular biologic techniques, we may gain insight in future studies.

REFERENCES

Epstein J, Xiao H, He X-Y (1990) Markers of multiple hematopoietic-cell lineages in multiple myeloma. N Engl J Med 322:664-668.

Garrett IR, Durie BGM, Nedwin GE, Gillespie A, Bringman T, Sabatina M, Bertolini DR, Mundy GR (1987) Production of lymphotoxin, a bone-resorbing cytokine, by cultured human myeloma cells. N Engl J Med 317:526-532.

Ho M, Miller G, Atchison RW, Breinig MK, Dummer JS, Andiman W, Starzl TE, Eastman R, Griffin BP, Hardesty RL, Bahnson T, Hakala TR, Rosenthal JT (1985) Epstein-Barr virus infections and DNA hybridization studies in posttransplantation lymphoma and lymphoproliferative lesions: The role of primary infection. J Infect Dis 152:876-886.

Hoover RN. Epidemiological evidence of tumor promotion (unpublished conference proceeding).

Jacobson DR, Zolla-Pazner S (1986) Immunosuppression and infection in multiple myeloma. Semin Oncol 13:282-290.

List AF, Greco A, Vogler LB (1987) Lymphoproliferative diseases in immunocompromised hosts: The role of Epstein-Barr virus. J Clin Oncol 5:1673-1689.

MacKenzie M, Lewis JP (1985) Cytogenetic evidence that the malignant event in multiple myeloma occurs in a precursor lymphocyte. Cancer Genet Cytogenet 17:13-20.

[2] J. Carney was responsible for data analyses.

MacKenzie MR, Paglieroni TG, Warner NL (1987) Multiple myeloma: An immunologic profile IV. The EA rosette-forming cell is a Leu-1 positive immunoregulatory B-cell. J Immunol 139:24-28.
Mueller N, Evans, A, Harris NL, Comstock GW, Jellum E, Magnus K, Orentreich N, Polk BF, Vogelman J (1989) Hodgkin's disease and EBV: Altered antibody pattern before diagnosis. N Eng J Med 320:696-701.
Mueller N, Evans AS, London T (1990) Viruses. In Schottenfeld D, Fraumeni JF Jr. (eds) *Cancer Epidemiology and Prevention.* Second Edition, Oxford University Press, New York (In press).
Selvanayagam P, Blick M, Narni F, van Tuinen P, Ledbetter D, Alexanian R, Saunders GF, Barlogie B (1988) Alteration and abnormal expression of the C-myc oncogene in human multiple myeloma. Blood 71:30-35.
Yoshida M, Seiki M, Yamaguchi K, Takasuki K(1984) Monoclonal integration of HTLV in all primary tumors of adult T-cell leukemia suggests causative role of HTLV in the disease. Proc Natl Acad Sci USA 81:2534-2537.

Clinical Studies

Biology of Multiple Myeloma - An Overview

Bart Barlogie, M.D.

University of Arkansas for Medical Sciences
301 W. Markham, Slot 508
Little Rock, Arkansas 72205

INTRODUCTION

Multiple myeloma (MM) is rapidly emerging as a new model of human neoplastic disease, after decades of limited interest by laboratory investigators in part because of its relatively low incidence and often indolent clinical course. Novel concepts in therapy, including effective salvage therapy with the VAD regimen (Barlogie 1984), high dose and even marrow-ablative therapy requiring hemopoietic stem cell support (Barlogie 1987; Gahrton 1987; Fermand 1989), and interferon for early and low tumor mass disease (Mellstedt 1979; Mandelli 1988), have all drawn new attention to human MM that affects mainly the elderly (median age, 65 years), more males (male to female ratio 1.5) and an increasing number of black patients, at least in the United States. While regularly inducible in murine species with pristane oil (Potter 1986), etiology and pathogenesis of human MM have remained obscure.

This chapter summarizes the results of recent laboratory investigation into the cellular and molecular biology of human MM, in order to provide a framework for future studies, especially those likely to shed further light on the etiology of this currently incurable human malignancy.

MYELOMA GENOTYPE

Laboratory studies in leukemia and lymphoma have revealed clearly that disease manifestations and prognosis can be defined most succinctly by specific chromosomal and molecular anomalies. Owing to the typically low proliferative activity of the predominant mature plasma cell phenotype with a median labelling index of one percent, cytogenetic information is sparse. Unlike cytogenetic studies, requiring cell cycle progression of tumor cells into mitosis, diagnosis of aneuploidy by nuclear DNA analysis is typically based on cells with a G-1 DNA complement and is thus proliferation-independent. Fortunately, nuclear DNA content abnormalities have been observed in about 80% of many hundreds of patients with MM as well as in about one-half of those with monoclonal gammopathy of unknown significance (MGUS), which represents most likely an important precursor condition to overt MM (Barlogie 1989A). Nuclear DNA content abnormalities, as determined conveniently by flow cytometry with appropriate fluorescent dyes, are usually of the hyperdiploid variety with an average DNA excess of 15%; only about 5 to 10% of patients present with hypodiploid DNA stem lines associated with secretion of Bence-Jones protein only and with absolute refractoriness to standard doses of chemotherapy (Barlogie 1985B). Hypodiploid abnormalities appear to prevail among the rare patients presenting under age 30.

Concurrent analysis of cellular RNA content and especially of cytoplasmic immunoglobulin together with nuclear DNA (see below) revealed the occasional presence of 2 tumor cell DNA stem lines (15%)

(Barlogie 1985A). As with hypodiploid abnormalities, such DNA-biclonal disease likewise has been found to be associated with resistance to primary therapy (Smith 1986).

Nuclear DNA abnormalities represent a stable stigma of an individual patient's MM over the entire time course of the disease process. In case of extramedullary disease presentation, over 80% of patients demonstrate concordant DNA patterns in bone marrow and extramedullary sites. Circulating DNA-aneuploid cells can be detected at a low frequency of up to 5% in about one-half of some 50 patients studied carefully, regardless of their stage of disease (Barlogie 1989A).

In addition to technical difficulties in obtaining a sufficient quantity of metaphases and at variance with well-defined nuclear DNA abnormalities, cytogenetic studies reveal highly complex karyotype aberrations, consisting of extensive chromosomal gains and deletions along with chromosomal breaks and translocations, many of which occur all within the same metaphase. Most investigators consider chromosomal translocations as the primary genetic lesion, whereas numeric anomalies are felt to represent secondary changes associated with disease evolution. The complexity of chromosomal aberrations is most consistent with a long disease latency prior to clinical diagnosis, as suggested by a long 20 year time interval between the nuclear fall out from the atomic bomb and disease manifestations of MM. Likewise, the transition from MGUS to overt MM occurs with a frequency per year of about 1% with cumulative frequencies of 10 and 20% after 10 and 20 years, respectively (Kyle 1984).

Among the cytogenetic abnormalities reported, there are chromosomal translocations resembling those observed in non-Hodgkin lymphoma such as t(11;14), t(14;18) and t(8;14) (Barlogie 1989A). Such translocations were typically associated with an IgA isotype. Ideogram analysis showed clustering of chromosomal breakpoints on the short arm of chromosome 1 band p11, on chromosome 8 near q24 (the location of c-myc), on the short arm of chromosome 11 and on chromosome 14 q32 (the site of the immunoglobulin heavy chain gene). These and other studies all do suggest a frequent occurrence of structural chromosomal aberrations and most likely translocations, although the chromosome partners are often not identified, in part due to relatively poor chromosomal morphology in MM.

Major advances in MM cytogenetics can be expected from the application of recently identified growth factors, especially IL-6, IL-3 and GM-CSF (Kawano 1988; Klein 1989A; Klein 1989B). When combined with high resolution chromosome banding studies and immunophenotype studies to trace a given chromosomal anomaly to either a myeloma tumor cell or normal hemopoietic elements (Knuutila 1989), myeloma-specific chromosomal lesions will hopefully be identified more readily and frequently in the future. The occasional presence of monosomy 5 or 7 may be related to a coincident myelodysplastic syndrome, as a result of cytotoxic therapy, or to the myeloma disease process itself. Considering the likely evolution of MM from a MGUS-type state, major efforts should be dedicated to identify chromosomal anomalies in MGUS, as they may represent the earlier genetic lesion, on the background of which the greater complexity of aberrations in MM evolves.

At this time, some associations between karyotype abnormalities and disease manifestation have been elucidated including the aforementioned prevalence of an IgA isotype among lymphoma-like translocations, drug resistance with a hypodiploid modal chromosome number, osteolytic bone disease with 6 q- abnormalities (site of TNF-beta as the major osteoclast-activating factor), and multi-drug resistance with chromosome 7q aberration (Barlogie 1989A).

ONCOGENES IN MYELOMA

Studies of the potential role of cellular oncogenes have been guided by cytogenetic anomalies in lymphoma and leukemia. In the absence of myeloma-specific chromosomal aberrations, oncogene studies were frequently initiated on the basis of rather vague cytogenetic observations. Because of its role in murine plasma-cytoma and supported by the occasional observation of Burkitt-type translocations [t(8;14) (q 24; q 32)], much of the initial work has focused on the c-myc oncogene (Selvanayagam 1988; Sumegi 1985; Meltzer 1987). While rearrangements of c-myc are the exception and usually different from those reported previously in lymphoma, myc-RNA is often strongly expressed in about one-quarter of patients examined carefully (Selvanayagam 1988). Examination of other cellular genes associated with B-cell lymphoma revealed bcl-1 rearrangement in only 5 of 120 patients examined (Selvanayagam 1987), concordant with the rare frequency of the t(11;14) translocation, which is more frequently observed in chronic lymphocytic leukemia. Although t(14;18) translocations typical of follicular lymphoma have occasionally been observed in plasma cell myeloma, rearrangement of the bcl-2 gene could not be demonstrated among 60 myeloma bone marrow samples (Barlogie 1989A). It is conceivable, however, that the use of high resolution banding techniques and pulse field electrophoresis both will lead to a more frequent observation of bcl-2 gene involvement in plasma cell myeloma as well. The Philadelphia chromosome has been reported in a single human myeloma cell line (Carpas 1982) but, to our knowledge, never in fresh clinical samples, although the recent notion of plasma cell myeloma as a stem cell malignancy would make such genetic abnormality rather attractive (Epstein 1990). Molecular studies have not yet been performed to determine whether submicroscopic Philadelphia-like gene rearrangements resulting in bcr-abl fusion products occur in clinical samples from MM patients.

PHENOTYPE

Consistent with the commitment of mature plasma cells to protein production, cellular RNA levels are markedly elevated, on average 6-fold compared to circulating lymphocytes, as appreciated on flow cytometric examination with the metachromatic dye acridine orange (Latreille 1980). The hallmark of plasma cells, monoclonal cytoplasmic immunoglobulin, is present in almost all patients with MM except the occasional case with non-producing disease (Barlogie 1985A). About 15% reveal kappa and lambda light chain co-expression, while the remaining 85% have either kappa or lambda light chain restriction upon examination with appropriate antisera. The apparent violation of the dogma of light chain isotype restriction was also confirmed by molecular analysis in a few instances where both kappa and lambda light chain genes were rearranged. Even more surprising was the occasional germ line expression of both heavy and light chain genes in sufficiently enriched tumor cell populations; in such cases, rearrangements of TCR-gamma and TCR-delta genes were also demonstrated (Lee 1987).

A systematic analysis of surface marker expression in multiple myeloma by several investigators showed the presence of the pre-B-cell antigen Calla+ in about 50% (Caligaris-Cappio 1985; Epstein 1988), of T and NK cell antigens (Van Camp 1990) as well as myelomonocytic (Grogan 1989), erythroid and even megakaryocytic markers in over 50% in some 30 to 50 cases (Epstein 1990). These observations have led Epstein *et al* to postulate that plasma cell myeloma may originate at a very early stage in hemopoietic development and lead, as a result of a relaxed differentiation program, to the expression of markers unusual for the normal stage of terminal B-cell differentiation, often in association with the typical plasma cell phenotype (cytoplasmic immunoglobulin) (Epstein 1990). This hypothesis has found its critics, arguing that the origin from a pluripotent stem cell in myeloma was incompatible with the observed clonal B-cell expansion. Perhaps, a series of initiating and promoting events are actually operating, explaining the infrequent and usually late progression from monoclonal gammopathy of unknown significance (MGUS) to overt plasma cell myeloma.

GROWTH FACTORS AND RECEPTORS

Investigations performed in several laboratories, mainly by Klein and Bataille (Klein 1989A) and by Caligaris-Cappio (F Caligaris-Cappio, unpublished observations), have established that the original demonstration by Kawano and co-workers of an autocrine interleukin-6 growth mechanism is probably the exception (Kawano 1988). Instead, bone marrow monocytes and macrophages seem to be the source of IL-6 triggering DNA synthesis and proliferation in neighboring myeloma plasma cells. Stimulation *in vitro* of human myeloma cells by IL-6 seems to be possible only when tumor cell proliferative activity is already high *in vivo*. *In vitro* growth adaptation requires an initial phase with GM-CSF or IL-3 in most cases before responsiveness to IL-6 can be observed. Collectively, IL-6 seems to be the primary growth factor in myeloma, operating through a paracrine mechanism in most instances, with monocytes and macrophages serving as the primary sources. The production by tumor cells of TNF-beta (Garrett 1987) and IL-1-beta (Kawano 1989; Carpas 1982), exerting osteoclast-activating activity, may stimulate normal accessory cells, especially monocytes and macrophages, to produce IL-6, GM-CSF and IL-3, which in turn have direct and/or indirect effects on plasma cell proliferation, mediated through specific receptors. The role of the bone marrow stroma in supporting tumor cell growth is also undergoing active investigation (F Caligaris-Cappio, unpublished observations). Whether osteoclasts, thought be derived from CFU-GM, may be part of the neoplastic clone is also being scrutinized. The role of IL-6 has already found clinical application, in that its serum levels seem to reflect tumor mass and disease activity (Bataille 1989). Soluble IL-6 receptor molecules have not yet been demonstrated, although an analogy should exist with the IL-2-receptor where the serum concentration of s-IL-2-R reflects tumor mass in CLL and hairy cell disease (Zambello 1989; Ambrosetti 1989). The eminent roles of IL-6 and IL-6-R in myeloma have already prompted clinical trials with anti-IL-6 monoclonal antibody, showing biological activity in 2 patients treated to date (B Klein, personal communication). It is conceivable that an immunotoxin approach with IL-6 linked to diphtheria toxin or ricin-A chain may lead to tumor cell inactivation upon binding to the IL-6-receptor on tumor cells. Whether or not this approach is sufficiently selective depends on the presence, intensity, and affinity of IL-6-R to IL-6 on normal host cells.

FUTURE CLUES FROM CLINICAL INVESTIGATION

The most pressing issue is to intensify cytogenetic studies and apply them to individuals with MGUS as a potential precursor condition of plasma cell myeloma. This will entail the utilization of a variety of growth factors in order to stimulate and expand a putative tumor precursor cell that may bear the primary genetic lesion in MM. A second area of great interest is the scrutinous examination of patients who have undergone allogeneic or autologous bone marrow transplantation and who are followed with low levels of disease activity, often for several years, before relapse ensues. This provides the clinical investigator and laboratory scientist with the unique opportunity to capture the very evolutionary steps that may occur during the natural development of the disease from MGUS. Thirdly, the provocative concept of myeloma as an early hemopoietic stem cell disorder with a benign phase of MGUS followed by an accelerated disease, multiple myeloma, and finally terminating in a high grade disease with high LDH (Barlogie 1989B), has many analogies to chronic myelocytic leukemia, where the molecular lesion has been defined and the bcr-abl product linked pathogenetically to the disease process by elegant retroviral transduction experiments (Lugo 1990). It is anticipated that similar research in MM will bridge the gap to the mouse model where a progression from an oil granuloma to autonomous plasma cell proliferation has been associated with activation of c-myc and a number of other cellular genes (Potter 1986).

REFERENCES

Ambrosetti A, Semenzato G, Prior M, Chilosi M, Vinante F, Vincenzi C, Zanotti R, Trentin L, Portuese A, Menestrina F, .et al (1989) Serum levels of soluble interleukin-2 receptor in hairy cell leukaemia: a reliable marker of neoplastic bulk. Br J Haematol: 181

Barlogie B, Alexanian R, Dicke K, Zagers G, Spitzer G, Jagannath S, Horwitz L (1987) High dose chemoradiotherapy and autologous bone marrow transplantation for resistant multiple myeloma. Blood 70:869

Barlogie B, Alexanian R, Pershouse M, Smallwood L, Smith L (1985A) Cytoplasmic immunoglobulin content in multiple myeloma. J Clin Invest 76:765

Barlogie B, Alexanian R, Smith L, Dixon D, Smallwood L, Delasalle K (1985B) Prognostic implications of tumor cell DNA and RNA, content in multiple myeloma. Blood 66:338

Barlogie B, Epstein J, Selvanayagam P, Alexanian R (1989A) Review Article: Plasma cell myeloma - new biological insights and advances in therapy. Blood 73:865

Barlogie B, Smallwood L, Smith T, Alexanian R (1989B) High serum levels of lactic dehydrogenase identify a high grade lymphoma-like myeloma. Ann Intern Med 110:521

Barlogie B, Smith L, Alexanian R (1984) Effective treatment of advanced multiple myeloma refractory to alkylating agents. N Engl J Med 310:1353

Bataille R, Jourdan M, Zhang XG, Klein B (1989) Serum levels of interleukin-6, a potent myeloma cell growth factor, as a reflect of disease severity in plasma cell dyscrasias. J Clin Inves 84:2008

Caligaris-Cappio F, Bergui L, Tesio L, Pizzolo G, Malavasi F, Chilosi M, Campana D, van Camp B, Jonossy G (1985) Identification of malignant plasma cell precursors in the bone marrow of multiple myeloma. J Clin Invest 76:1243

Carpas A, Fischer P, Swirsky D (1982) Human myeloma cell line carrying a Philadelphia Chromosome. Sci 216:997

Cozzolino F, Torcia M, Aldinucci D, Ruibartelli A, Miliani A, Shaw R, Lansdorp AR, Di Guglielmo R (1989) Production of interleukin-1 by bone marrow myeloma cells: Its role in the pathogenesis of lytic bone lesions. Blood 74:380

Epstein J, Barlogie B, Katzmann J, Alexanian R (1988) Phenotypic heterogeneity in aneuploid multiple myeloma indicates pre-B cell involvement. Blood 71:861

Epstein J, Huiqing X, Xiao-Yan H (1990) Markers of multiple hematopoietic-cell lineages in multiple myeloma. N Eng J Med 322:664

Fermand JP, Levy Y, Gerota J, Benbunan M, Cosset JM, Castaigne S, Seligmann M, Brouet JC (1989) Treatment of agressive multiple myeloma by high-dose chemotherapy and total body irradiation followed by blood stem cell autologous grafts. Blood 73:20

Gahrton G, Tura S, Flesch M, Gratwohl A, Gravett P, Lucarelli G,

Michallet M, Reiffers J, Ringden O, van Lint MT, Vernant JP, Zwaan FE (1987) Bone marrow transplantation in multiple myeloma. Report from the European Cooperative Group for Bone Marrow Transplantation. Blood 69:126

Garrett LR, Durie BGM, Nedwin GE, Gillespie A, Bringman T, Sabatini M, Bertolini DR, Mundy GR (1987) Production of the bone resorbing cytokine lymphotoxin by cultures human myeloma cells. N Engl J Med 317:526

Grogan TM, Durie BGM, Spier CM, Richter L, Vela E (1989) Myelomonocytic antigen positive multiple myeloma. Blood 73:763

Kawano M, Hirano T, Matsuda T, Taga T, Horii Y, Iwato K, Asaoku H, Tang B, Tanabe O, Tanaka H, Kuramoto A, Kishimoto T (1988) Autocrine generation and requirement of BSF-2/IL-6 for human multiple myelomas. Nature 332:83

Kawano M, Yamamoto I, Iwato K, Tanaka H, Asaoku H, Tanabe O, Ishikawa H, Nobuyoshi M, Ohmoto Y, Hirai Y, et al (1989) Interleukin-1 beta rather than lymphotoxin as the major bone resorbing activity in human multiple myeloma. Blood 73:1646

Klein B, Zhang X-G, Jourdan M, Bataille R (1989A) GM-CSF synergizes with interleukin-6 in supporting the proliferation of human myeloma cells. Blood 74:749A

Klein B, Zhang X-G, Jourdan M, Content J, Houssiau F, Aarden L, Piechaczyk M, Bataille R (1989B) Paracrine rather than autocrine regulation of myeloma-cell growth and differentiation by interleukin-6. Blood 73:517

Knuutila S, Teerenhovi L (1989) Immunophenotyping of aneuploid cells. Cancer Genet Cytogenet 41:1-17

Kyle, RA (1984) "Benign" monoclonal gammopathy: A misnomer? JAMA 251:1849

Latreille J, Barlogie B, Gohde W, Johnston D, Drewinko B, Alexanian R (1980) Cellular DNA content as a marker of human multiple myeloma. Blood 55:403

Lee M, Selvanayagam P, Alexanian R, Stass S, Barlogie B (1987) Rearrangement (REARR) of T-cell receptor (TCR) gamma chain gene in multiple myeloma. AACR, Abstract #706

Lugo T, Pendegast AM, Muller A, Witte O (1990) Tyrosine kinase activity and transformation potency of bcr-abl oncogene products. Sci 247:1009

Mandelli F, Tribalto M, Avvisati G, Cantonetti M, Petrucci M, Boccadoro M, Pileri A, Marmont F, Resengotti L, Lauta V, Dammacco F (1988) Recombinant interferon alfa-2b (Intron A) as post-induction therapy for responding multiple myeloma patients. M84 protocol. Cancer Treat Rev (suppl A):43

Mellstedt H, Ahre A, Bjorkholm M, Holm G, Johansson B, Strander H (1979) Interferon therapy in myelomatosis. Lancet 1:245

Meltzer P, Shadle K, Durie B (1987) Somatic mutation alters a critical region of the c-myc gene in multiple myeloma. Blood 70:985A

Potter M (1986) Plasmacytomas in mice. Semin Oncol 13:275

Selvanayagam P, Blick M, Narni F, Van Tuinen P, Ledbetter D, Alexanian R, Saunders G, Barlogie B (1988) Alteration and abnormal expression of the c-myc oncogene in human multiple myeloma. Blood 71:30

Selvanayagam P, Goodacre A, Strong L, Saunders G, Barlogie B (1987) Alterations of bcl-1 oncogene in human multiple myeloma. AACR, Abstract #76

Smith L, Barlogie B, Alexanian R (1986) Biclonal and hypodiploid multiple myeloma. Am J Med 80:841

Sumegi J, Hedberg T, Bjorkholm M, Godal T, Mellstedt H, Nilsson MG, Perlman C, Klein G (1985) Amplification of the c-myc oncogene in human plasma cell leukemia. Int J Cancer 36:367

Van Camp B, Durie BGM, Spier C, De Waele M, Van Reit I, Vela E, Frutiger Y, Richter L, Grogan TM (In Press) Plasma cells in multiple myeloma express a natural killer cell associated antigen CD 56 [NKH-1; Leu-19]. Blood: July 15, 1990

Zambello R, Pizzolo G, Trentin L, Agostini C, Chisesi T, Vinante F, Scarselli E, Zanotti R, De Rossi G, et al (1989) Evaluation of serum levels of soluble interleukin-2 receptor in patients with chronic lymphoproliferative disorders of T-lymphocytes. Cancer: 2019

Open Discussion on the Biology of Multiple Myeloma. Chairman's Introductory Remarks

Kenneth Nilsson

Laboratory of Tumor Biology, Department of Pathology, University of Uppsala, S-751 85 Uppsala, Sweden

INTRODUCTION

As a background for this discussion on the biology of multiple myeloma (MM) I will make a few remarks about the pathogenesis of the disease and the role of interleukin-6 (IL-6) as a growth factor for MM cells. I will finally argue that, since IL-6 stimulates the growth of MM cells by a paracrine rather than an autocrine mechanism, knowledge about the regulation of the IL-6 production in the non-MM bone-marrow cells may be relevant for epidemiological studies on MM.

ASPECTS ON THE PATHOGENESIS OF MM

The following basic facts about the pathogenesis of MM may serve as a basis for a hypothetical discussion on the development of MM:

1. As suggested by clinical data and cytogenetic studies the development of MM appears to be a multi-step process during which successive, multiple and alternative (?) genetic changes of the transforming target cell(s) lead to a gradual independence of normal control mechanisms for growth and differentiation.

2. The nature of the target cell of the malignant transformation is not known. However, since the immunoglobulin (Ig) genes are rearranged in MM it should be a B-cell and not a cell of the pluri-or multipotent hematopoietic stem cell compartments or a pro-B cell.

3. The cytogenetic changes are heterogeneous and complex (Liang et al 1979; Philip 1980; Lewis and MacKenzie 1984; Dewald et al 1985; Jernberg et al 1987; Gould et al 1988). They include numerical aberrations, gains (# 1,3,5,7,9,11,14), losses (8,13), translocations (t(8;14; t(11;14), t(14;18), t(14;?)) and deletions. It may be significant that the break on chromosome 14 most frequently occurs in the Ig heavy chain locus (14q32). Rearrangements of c-*myc* and *bcl*-1 are rare (Selvanayagam et al 1988). Mutations of *ras* oncogenes (predominantly N-*ras*, but also H-*ras* and K-*ras*) were found in about 30% (Neri et al 1989).

3. The cause of the genetic changes is unknown. Excessive expansion of one or several B-cell clones, due to antigenic stimulation and/or defective T-cell control of antigen responses, has been suggested to

represent a pre-neoplastic event. Imperfect repair of alterations in genes associated with growth control, occurring "spontaneously" as a consequence of such an increased proliferation, may also represent an important step in the evolution of an MM.

4. The resultant malignant, clinically detectable, MM clone will continue to undergo genetic changes (progression), which may be associated with further alterations of its clinical behaviour (e.g. growth rate, Ig synthesis, osteolysis, immune suppression and response to therapy).

5. Like chronic myelogeneous leukemia (CML) MM seems to represent a hematopoietic malignancy with ongoing differentiation. The knowledge about the nature of the putative, circulating blood "stem cells" is fragmentary.

GROWTH FACTORS FOR MM CELLS

Over the last 2 years it has been demonstrated that about 40-60% of MM biopsy cells and MM cell lines respond to IL-6 stimulation (Kawano et al 1988; Klein et al 1989; Anderson et al 1989; Nilsson 1989; Tanabe et al 1989; Shimizu et al 1989; Nilsson et al 1990). Furthermore, autocrine IL-6 production seems to be rare as judged by studies on IL-6 mRNA expression by northern blot analysis and IL-6 protein production using bio- and radioimmunoassays (Klein et al 1989; Nilsson 1989).

For normal B-cells IL-6 appears to be a differentiation-and not a growth factor (Kishimoto 1989). It has therefore been speculated that an important defect in MM cells is the deranged response to IL-6 in that MM cells "misinterpret" the IL-6 signal as a growth and not a differentiation signal.

The growth regulation of IL-6 independent MM is unknown but studies on MM cell lines suggest that, as yet unidentified growth factors are produced suggesting the possibility of autocrine growth (Klein et al 1987).

For biopsy cells also IL-3, IL-5, IL-1 and GM-CSF may be growth stimulatory, often together with IL-6. In cell lines, however, only IL-6 is clearly growth promoting (Nilsson et al 1990). This leaves the possibility open that the stimulation of these factors observed in the biopsy cells, is indirect, via stimulation of non-MM bone marrow cells. Interestingly, interferon (IFN)α and IFNγ may affect the growth of MM cells (Klein et al to be published; Jernberg et al to be published). IFN γ inhibits the growth of IL-6 dependent MM biopsy cells and cell lines by an unknown mechanism. IFNα may stimulate proliferation at low concentrations but inhibits growth at high concentrations (Brenning 1985).

As has recently been shown for an MM cell line, U-266, the dependence on exogeneous IL-6 for growth can change towards independence (perhaps by the development of an autocrine loop) as a consequence of tumor progression (Nilsson et al 1990).

Myeloma cells produce several cytokines with the potential to stimulate non-MM bone marrow cells. Thus the production of IL-1ß, TNFα, TNFß, IGF-1 and TGFß has been suggested by studies on MM biopsy cells and cell lines. (reviewed by Nilsson et al 1990). Based on these studies, Fig.1 suggests a possible net-work type of interaction between MM cells and other bone-marrow cells with the potential for paracrine production of IL-6. In addition to the signalling between these cell types by hormonlike growth-and differentiation factors cell to cell contacts are important and appear to modify the response of the interacting cells to the different factors.

HYPOTHETICAL SCENARIOS FOR THE DEVELOPMENT OF MM

As pointed out before, the early stages of the development of MM are unknown, both with respect to target cell(s) and causation to the early genetic changes postulated to determine the deranged growth control typical of the clinical MM. However, based on the present knowledge one may speculate as follows:

Early genetic changes may lead to increased survival by deregulation of genes coding for "survival factors", e.g. *bcl-2*, or as yet unidentified genes responsible for the programmed cell death (apoptosis) of terminally differentiated B-cells. Such surviving cells may slowly proliferate and constitute the clinical picture of MGUS. The proliferation may be the result of IL-6 stimulation already at this early stage of MM development, but may also depend on other factors and cell-cell contacts. The evolution towards a more rapidly expanding tumor from MGUS would result from sequential genetic changes among MGUS cells, leading to the development of variant phenotypes within the expanding clone(s) and Darwinistic selection of cells with the fittest phenotype(s).

For the MM, which are IL-6 dependent at the time of diagnosis, the evolution of a proliferative response to IL-6 must be an important event if, as discussed, IL-6 normally is a differentiation factor. If, on the other hand, normal term nal B-cells are indeed induced to proliferation by IL-6 one woulu postulate that an important step in the MM evolution would be an increased production of IL-6 by the non-MM bone marrow cells.

For IL-6 independent MM IL-6 might have been an important growth factor earlier during the evolution to the clincally detectable tumor. However, in this case the IL-6 dependency was lost (as found for the U-266 MM cell line during long term culture) in favour of other, more powerful mechanisms of growth stimulation. Alternatively, IL-6 independent MM were never responsive to IL-6 throughout the whole period of evolution.

POSSIBLE CYTOKINE-NETWORK INTERACTIONS BETWEEN MM AND SOME CELL TYPES IN THE BONE MARROW

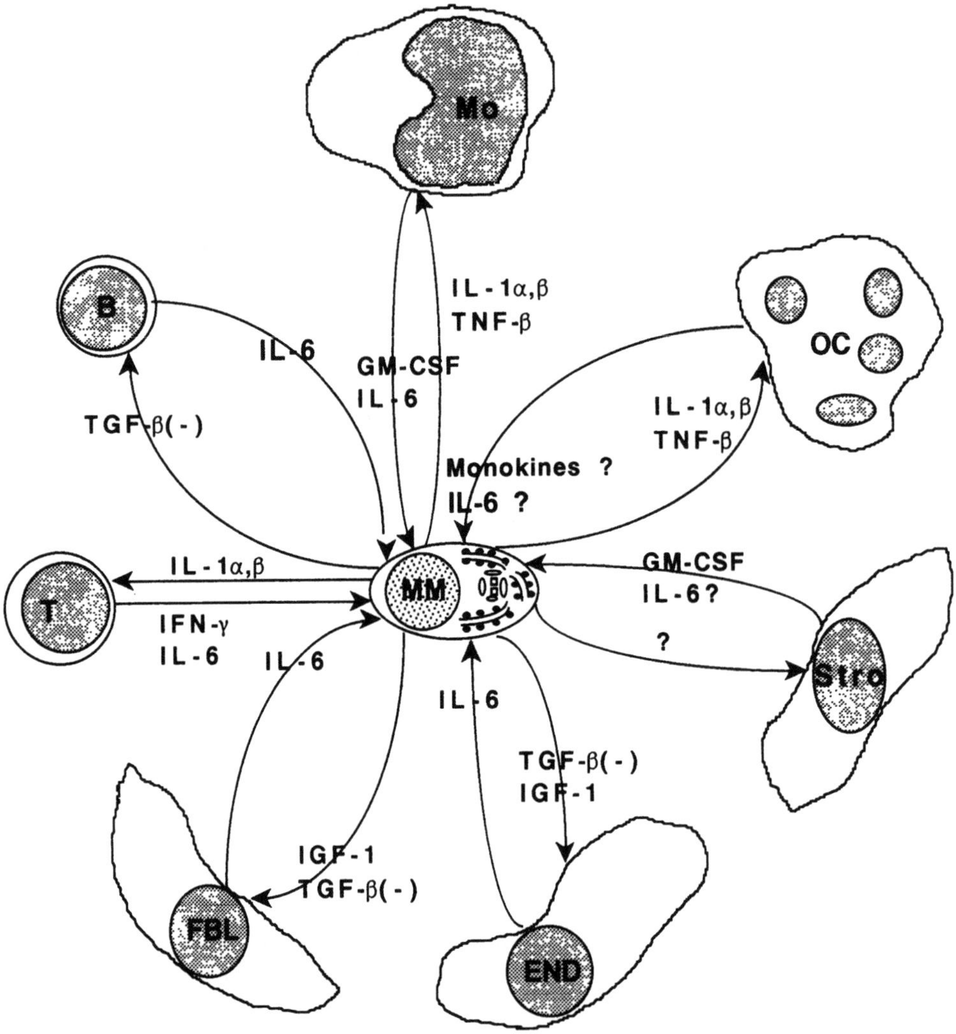

Fig.1 T=T cell; B = B cell; Mo = monocyte; OC = osteoclast; Stro = stromal cell; END = endothelial cell; FBL = fibroblast.

CONCLUSION

For studies on the epidemiology of myeloma the excistance of a paracrine IL-6 growth stimulation of a large fraction of MM seems to be interesting since it points to the possibility that environmental factors, which can stimulate IL-6 production in non-MM bone marrow cells may be etiologically important for the development of clinical MM. Such factors are unknown but, as inflammation is associated with IL-6 production (Kishimoto 1989), they include anything that stimulates and maintains an inflammatory response. (Van Damme et al 1989; Nemunaitis et al 1989; Jirik et al 1989). Viral infections might directly induce IL-6 production by activation of nuclear factor IL-6, which regulates the production of IL-6 (Akira et al 1990), and indirectly by inducing bone marrow cells to IL-6 production during an inflammatory response. Viral infections may also affect the growth of an MM clone by the induction of IFNα and IFNγ production, leading either to growth inhibition (high concentrations of IFNα and IFNγ) or perhaps even growth stimulation (low concentration of IFNα).

ACKNOWLEDGEMENTS

This work was supported by a grant from the Swedish Cancer Society. I thank Mrs Eva Harrysson for assistance in the preparation of this manuscript.

REFERENCES

Akira S, Isshiki H, Sugita T, Tanabe O, Kinoshita S, Nishio Y, Nakajima T, Hirano T, Kishimoto T (1990) A nuclear factor for IL-6 expression (NF-IL6) is a member of a C/EBP-family. EMBO J 9:1897-1906.
Andersson K C, Jones R M, Morimoto C, Leavitt P, Barut B A (1989) Response patterns of purified myeloma cells to hematopoietic growth factors. Blood 73:1915-1924.
Brenning G (1985) The *in vitro* effect of leukocyte-α interferon on human myeloma cells in a semisolid agar culture system. Scand J Haematol 35:178-185.
Dewald G W, Kyle R A, Hicks G A, Greipp P R (1985) The clinical significance of cytogenetic studies in 100 patients with multiple myeloma. Plasma cell leukemia, or amyloidosis. Blood 66:380-390.
Gould J, Alexanian R, Goodacre A, Pathak S, Hecht B, Barlogie B (1988) Plasma cell karyotype in multiple myeloma. Blood 71:453-456.
Jernberg H, Zech L, Nilsson K (1987) Cytogenetic studies on human myeloma cell lines. Int J Cancer 40:811-817.
Jirik F R, Podor T J, Hirano T, Kishimoto T, Loskutoff D J, Carson D A, Lots M (1989) Bacterial lipopolysaccharide and inflammatory mediators augment IL-6 secretion by human endothelial cells. J Immunol 142:144-147.
Kawano M, Hirano T, Matsuda T, Taga T, Horii Y, Iwato K, Asaoku H, Tang B, Tanabe O, Tanaka H, Kuramoto A, Kishimoto T (1988) Autocrine generation and requirement of BSF-2/IL-6 for human multiple myelomas. Nature 332:83-85.
Kishimoto T (1989) The biology of interleukin-6. Blood 74:1-10.

Klein B, Jourdan M, Vazques A, Dugas B, Bataille R (1987) Production of growth factors by human myeloma cells. Cancer Res 47:4856-4860.
Klein B, Zhang X-G, Jourdan M, Content J, Houssiau F, Aarden L, Piechaczyk M, Bataille R (1989) Paracrine rather than autocrine regulation of myeloma-cell growth and differentiation by interleukin-6. Blood 73:517-526.
Lewis J P, MacKenzie M R (1984) Non-random chromosomal aberrations associated with multiple myeloma. Hematol Oncol 2:307-317.
Liang W, Hopper J E, Rowley J D (1979) Karyotypic abnormalities and clinical aspects of patients with multiple myeloma and related paraproteinemic disorders. Cancer 44:630-644.
Nemunaitis J, Andres D F, Mochizuki D Y, Lilly M B, Singer J W (1989) Human marrow stromal cells: Response to interleukin-6 (IL-6) and control of IL-6 expression. Blood 74:1929-1935.
Neri A, Murphy J P, Cro L, Ferrero D, Tarella C, Baldini L, Dalla-Favera R (1989) *ras* oncogene mutation in multiple myeloma. J Exp Med 170:1715-1725.
Nilsson K (1989) IN: F Melchers, M Potter (eds.) Mechanisms of B cell neoplasia. Editiones Roche, Basel, Switzerland, pp 229-235.
Nilsson K, Jernberg H, Pettersson M (1990) IL-6 as a growth factor for human multiple myeloma cells - a short overview. IN: F Melchers, M Potter (eds.) Current Topics of Microbiology and Immunology. Springer Verlag Berlin-Heidelberg-New York-London-Paris-Tokyo, in press.
Philip P (1980) Chromosomes of monoclonal gammopathies. Cancer Genet Cytogenet 2:79-86.
Selvanayagam P, Blick M, Narni F, van Tuinen P, Ledbetter D H, Alexanian R, Saunders G F, Barlogie B (1988) Alteration and abnormal expression of the c-*myc* oncogene in human multiple myeloma. Blood 71:30-35.
Shimizu S, Yoshioka R, Hirose Y, Sugai S, Tachibana J, Konda S (1989) Establishment of two interleukin 6 (B cell stimulatory factor 2/interferon ß2)-dependent human bone marrow-derived myeloma cell lines. J Exp Med 169:339-344.
Tanabe O, Kawano M, Tanaka H, Iwato K, Asaoku H, Ishikawa H, Nobuyoshi M, Hirano T, Kishimoto T, Kuramoto A (1989) BSF-2/IL-6 does not augment Ig secretion but stimulates proliferation in myeloma cells. Am J Hematol 31:258-262.
Van Damme J, Schaafsma M R, Fibbe W E, Falkenburg J H F, Opdenakker G, Billiau A (1989) Simultaneous production of interleukin 6, interferon-ß and colony-stimulating activity by fibroblasts after viral and bacterial infection. Eur J Immunol 19:163-168.

In Vitro Studies Provide Evidence that Multiple Paracrine Loops may be Operating in Multiple Myeloma

F. Caligaris-Cappio, L. Bergui, G.L. Gaidano, F. Merico, M. Schena.

Dipartimento Scienze Biomediche Oncologia Umana, Cattedra Clinica Medica A, Via Genova 23, 10126 Torino, Italy.

INTRODUCTION

Multiple Myeloma (MM) is a B cell malignancy characterized by the bone marrow (BM) accumulation of monoclonal plasmacells. Different clinical and experimental evidences favour the view that in human MM, as in murine plasmacytoma, the disease may be disseminated by clonogenic plasmacell precursors circulating in the peripheral blood (PB). The disease is widespread to the axial skeleton by the time of diagnosis, while very few plasmacells are seen in the PB and their number becomes evident only in the terminal phases of the disease. PB lymphocytes expressing the relevant idiotype have been described and PB mononuclear cells (PBMC) may show a monoclonal immunoglobulin (Ig) gene rearrangement. Also, DNA-aneuploid cells have been detected in PB samples and several methods have been described to grow plasmacell colonies from PB. Finally, MM PBMC cultured in vitro in presence of IL3 and IL6 give rise to a variable proportion of monoclonal B cells. In this work we have asked two questions: 1) how can we investigate the presence of malignant plasmacell precursors in the PB of patients with MM ?; 2) why are these precursors selectively homing to the BM ? In order to address these questions we have used a threefold approach: a) PBMC from MM patients have been cultured in presence of different combinations of cytokines; b) PBMC from MM patients have been cultured in presence of autologous serum; c) long term culture of BM stromal cells have been established from MM patients and characterized.

MM PBMC cultured in presence of cytokines

PBMC were obtained from 16 patients with MM at diagnosis before the initiation of treatment and cultured in presence of IL3 (15 U/ml) and IL6 (1,000 U/ml). After 3 days 1,000 U/ml of IL6 were added to the cultures. In 14/16 cases, variable proportions of immunoblast-like B cells appeared at day 3 and of plasmacells at day 6, thus confirming that the synergistic activity of IL3 and IL6 may be able to stimulate MM circulating precursors. In 5/16 cases IL3,IL6-induced day 3 blasts expressed the CD10 antigen which was subsequently lost during the transition to the plasmacell stage. The appearance of CD10 antigen led us to investigate the significance of this molecule as a marker for MM clonogenic cells. We studied this problem with two experimental approaches. First, we stimulated PBMC from 3 normal subjects with pokeweed mitogen (PWM) to evaluate whether the mere activation of normal PB lymphocytes might trigger the expression of CD10. In all the cases studied, day 6 plasmablasts developing after PWM stimulation were CD10$^+$, thus indicating that normal B cells, upon activation, come through a stage where they express the CD10 antigen. These findings are the in vitro counterpart of the in vivo well known observation that germinal centre (GC) B blasts are CD10$^+$. Next, we cultured PBMC from 5 patients with MM in presence of IL7 reasoning that MM circulating precursors would proliferate in presence of IL7 if they were very close derivatives of the stem cell, while they would be IL7-unresponsive if of peripheral (e.g. GC) origin. IL7 (200-1,000 U/ml) was used alone or in combination with 1,000

U/ml IL6. After 6 days of culture, a percentage of 38 + 7% large blast cells were apparent. As shown in Table 1, these cells were $CD3^+$, most of them were $CD4^+$and expressed the CD25 antigen in a rather high proportion, while failed to increase the expression of HLA-DR. The proportion of $CD3^+$, $CD4^+$, $CD25^+$ cells was further increased by the co-stimulation of IL7 and IL6 (Table 1). Since MM circulating precursor are IL7-unresponsive and the expression of CD10 may be triggered by the simple activation of normal circulating B lymphocytes, we come to the conclusion that MM CD10 bearing cells are most likely of peripheral origin. The unexpected T cell response to the addition of IL7 in the culture confirms recent data on the ability of IL7 to stimulate pre-activated T cells from normal PB and indicates that pre-activated $CD4^+$ cells are circulating in the peripheral blood of patients with MM.

MM PBMC cultured in presence of autologous serum

The rationale of this approach was threefold. First, IL6 levels have been reported to be elevated in the sera of patients with aggressive MM. Second, short-term cultures (6 days) of MM PBMC revealed the presence of high number of monocytes which reacted with anti-IL6 MoAbs (Fig. 1). Third, as already mentioned, activated T cells are circulating in the PB of MM patients and preliminary studies with a biological assay have shown that IL3 and granulocyte macrophage-colony stimulating factor (GM-CSF) levels are increased in the sera of some MM patients. On these bases, we cultured PBMC from 7 patients with MM and 2 patients with monoclonal gammopathy of unknown significance (MGUS) in presence of RPMI medium supplemented with 20-30% autologous serum (AS). Half of the spent medium was replaced by fresh medium + AS every four days. After 30 days of culture, variable proportions of plasmacells (Table 2) were found clustering around IL6-producing macrophages (Fig. 2). These data indicate that high proportions of IL6 producing monocytes are circulating in the PB of MM patients and that these cells may play a role in the development of malignant plasmacells from their precursors.

MM BM stromal cells

Both macrophages and T cells are present in the BM microenvironment. A further BM population is represented by the stromal cells whose features, well known in the mouse, are rather obscure in man. BM aspirate was obtained from 11 patients with MM. Nucleated cells were purified on methilcellulose and cultured on coverslips in 24 well culture plates in presence of Dulbecco medium and 5% horse serum (HS). When a confluent layer of cells was observed after 5-7 weeks of culture at 37°C in presence of 5% CO2 the adherent cells were characterized. These cells were mostly fibroblasts mixed with 10-15% scattered macrophages: no endothelial cells (Factor VIII antigen positive) were observed. A small number of large multinucleated cells were present at the edge of the coverslip: these cells were positively stained with the tartrate-resistant acid phosphatase (TRAP) reaction, organized cytoskeletal F-actin in small podosomes located at the periphery of the cell and had the receptors for calcitonin thus fulfilling the major criteria for identifying osteoclasts. In the supernatant of 7 week stromal cell cultures high levels of IL-6 (O.10 - 3.7. ng/ml) were detected. In 10/11 cases no residual lymphocytes or plasmacells could be detected after 7 weeks of culture as evaluated by staining coverslip adherent cells with CD19, CD3, anti-IgG, M, A, k, λ antibodies (Abs). These BM stromal cell cultures are now used as feeder layers to evaluate their ability of supporting the growth and differentiation of circulating MM clonogenic cells.

CONCLUSIONS

In conclusion, our observations indicate that in the peripheral blood of MM patients monoclonal plasmacell precursors circulate together with activated T and accessory cell populations. It is not unreasonable to postulate that when plasmacell precursors arrive to the BM come into contact with IL6 producing BM stromal cells, activated T cells and IL6 producing monocytes. The physical interactions between these populations may trigger the interplay of different paracrine loops and provide the most suitable microenvironment for the entrappment, proliferation and final differentiation of MM precursor cells thus leading to the progression and dissemination of MM malignant clone.

Acknowledgements: This work was supported by A.I.R.C., Milano. The IL7 we used was a kind gift of IMMUNEX, Seattle, WA.

Table 1. PBMC from MM patients cultured for 6 days in presence of IL-7 or of IL-7 + IL6.

	Control %	IL-7 %	IL-7 + IL-6 %
CD3+, CD4+	60 ± 6	> 90 *	> 90*
CD3+, CD8+	27 ± 6	< 10 *	< 10*
CD3+, CD25+	5 ± 3	18 ± 5§*	29 ± 4§*
CD3+, HLA-DR+	3 ± 2	5 ± 2*	7 ± 3*

5 pts studied (2 x 10^6 cells / ml). § Normal control subjects (4): 6 + 2;
* These data refer to the CD3+ large blast-like cells (38 + 7%)
IL-7 = 1,000 U/ml at day 0; IL-6 = 1,000 U/ml added at day 3.

Table 2. PBMC from MM and MGUS cultured in vitro in presence of autologous serum.

Isotype	Stage	PC (light chain) %*
Gk	III	25 (k: λ =7:1)
Gλ	III	20 (λ)
Gk	III	15 (k)
Gλ	III	1 (λ)
Ak	II	10 (k)
Gk	II	1 (k)
Gk	I	7 (k)
Gk	MGUS	0
Gk	MGUS	0
Normal controls (4)		0

* PC: plasmacells; percentage of monoclonal PC after 30 days of culture;

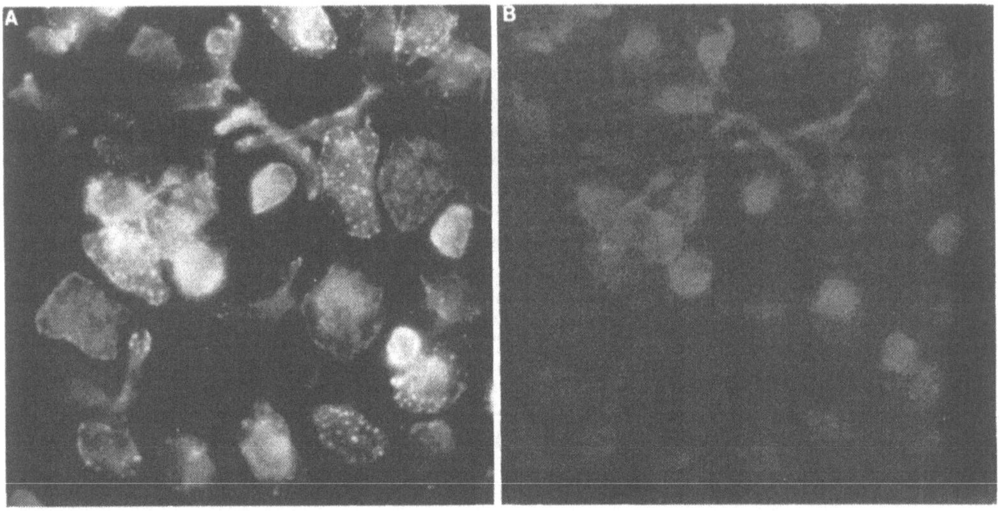

Fig. 1. High numbers of monocytes (revealed with an anti-F-actin Ab, panel A) are circulating in the PB of MM patients and react with anti-IL6 Abs (B).

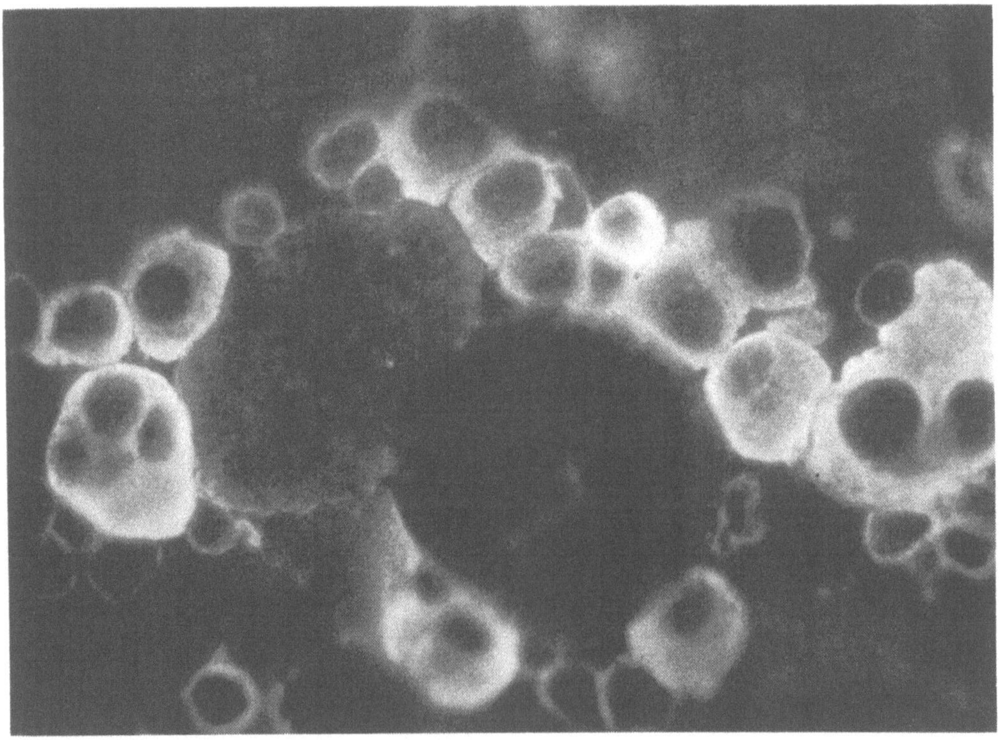

Fig. 2. Monoclonal lymphocytes and plasmacells growing around macrophages.

REFERENCES

Armitage RJ, Namen AE, Sassenfeld HM, Grabstein KH (1990) Regulation of human T cell proliferattion by IL-7. J Immunol 144:938-941.

Barlogie B, Epstein J, Selvanayagam P, Alexanian R (1989) Plasma cell myeloma - new biological insights and advances in therapy. Blood 73:865-873.

Barton B E, Mayer R (1989) IL-3 induces differentiation of bone marrow precursor cells to osteclast-like cells. J Immunol 143: 3211-3215.

Berenson J, Wong R, Kim K, Brown N, Lichstentein A (1987) Evidence of peripheral blood B lymphocyte but not T lymphocyte involvement in multiple myeloma. Blood. 70:1550-1553.

Bergui L, Schena M, Gaidano GL, Riva M, Caligaris-Cappio F (1989) Interleukin 3 and interleukin 6 synergistically promote the proliferation and differentiation of malignant plasma cell precursors in Multiple Myeloma. J Exp Med 170:613-618.

Durie, BGM, Salmon SE (1975) A clinical staging system for multiple myeloma. Cancer 36:842-854.

Hamburger, A.W., and S.E. Salmon. 1977 Primary bioassay of human myeloma stem cells. J. Clin. Invest. 60:846-854.

Kawano M, Hirano T, Matsuda T, Taga T, Horii Y, Iwato K, Asaoku H, Tang B, Tanabe O, Tanaka H, Kuramoto A, Kishimoto T (1988) Autocrine generation and requirement of BSF-2/IL-6 for human multiple myeloma. Nature 332:83-85.

Klein B, Zhang XG, Jourdan M, Content J, Houssiau F, Aarden L, Piechaczyk M, Bataille R (1989) Paracrine rather than autocrine regulation of Myeloma-cell growth and differentiation by interleuchin-6. Blood 73:517-526.

Kubagawa H, Vogler CB, Capra JD, Conrad ME, Lawton AR, Cooper MD (1979) Studies on the clonal origin of multiple myeloma. J Exp Med 150:792.

Mellstedt H, Hammarstrom S, Holm G (1974) Monoclonal lymphocyte population in human plasma cell myeloma. Clin Exp Immunol 17:371-376.

Nordan RP, Potter M (1986) A macrophage derived factor required by plasmacytomas for survival and proliferation in vitro. Science 233:566-569.

The Origin of Bone Marrow Plasma Cells

I.C.M. MacLennan and E.Y.T. Chan

Department of Immunology, University of Birmingham Medical School, Birmingham, B15 2TT, England.

INTRODUCTION

Myelomatosis is a neoplasm of bone marrow plasma cells, which characteristically does not involve other sites of antibody production such as the gut [Leonard et al 1979]. It is also a feature of the disease that the malignant plasma cells are usually committed to IgG or IgA production while IgM-producing myelomatosis almost never occurs (4 of 1651 consecutive patpatients entered into MRC myelomatosis trials).

These features coincide with those of physiological bone marrow plasma cells arising from B cells activated within the spleen or the peripheral lymph nodes during the established phase of T cell-dependent antibody responses [Benner et al 1981]. This paper describes the characteristics of these plasma cells and their progenitors and discusses the stages during B cell differentiation where genetic changes leading to neoplastic transformation may occur.

B CELLS ACTIVATED AT DIFFERENT SITES GIVE RISE TO PLASMA CELLS WITH DIFFERENT PROPERTIES

Three distinct types of microenvironment can be identified where B cells can be activated to give rise to plasma cells [MacLennan et al 1988 and 1990]. These are: (i) tissues where there are accumulations of macrophages; (ii) the areas of secondary lymphoid organs rich in T cells and interdigitating cells and (iii) the B cell follicles, which are found in all secondary lymphoid tissues.

Macrophage-associated B cell activation is the hall mark of responses to the T cell-independent type 1 (TI-1) antigens based on bacterial lipopolysaccharide (LPS) [Corbel and Melchers 1983]. Macrophages and many B cells have receptors for LPS [Smith et al 1979 and Levit et al 1981]. The combination of B cells and macrophages with TI-1 antigen appears to be sufficient to evoke antigen-specific B cell proliferation and differentiation to plasma cells. In studies of anti-hapten antibody responses to hapten-LPS conjugates, proliferation of hapten-specific B cells can be seen in macrophage-rich tissues such as the red pulp of the spleen [Zhang, Liu and MacLennan previously unpublished data]. B cells activated in this situation differentiate to become plasma cells in the same site. These plasma cells have a life-span in the order of three days [Ho et al 1986]. The secretion of any of the immunoglobulin classes may result; but it is significant that IgM production is a feature of B cell activation in association with macrophages. Most IgM-producing plasma cells in rat bone marrow, have a 3 day life span [Ho et al 1986]. It seems likely that they are generated by this type of B cell activation.

B cell activation in areas of secondary lymphoid tissue rich in T cells and interdigitating cells occurs in responses to T cell-dependent (TD) and TI-1 antigens during the first few days following exposure to antigen [MacLennan et al 1988 and 1990]. On secondary exposure to these classes of antigen the response in T zones may be very impressive, in terms of the number of antigen-specific B blasts, but the duration of the response is still only a matter of 3-4 days from secondary antigenic challenge. B cell proliferation occurs in T zones in response to T cell-independent type 2 antigens (TI-2) based on a pure polysaccharide core structure. B cell activation in T zones can continue for extended periods following exposure to these antigens. Available evidence suggests that these TI-2 responses are maintained by continued recruitment of virgin B cells into the response rather than memory B cell production [Lane et al 1986]. As in macrophage-associated B cell activation, one of any of the classes of immunoglobulin may be produced by plasma cells generated in T zones. Their life-span is again in the order of 3 days. The B cells activated in T zones, however, migrate to adjacent sites before becoming plasma cells. B cell activation in the T cell-rich periarteriolar lymphocytic sheaths of the spleen pass to the red pulp before becoming plasma cells. Those activated in the paracortex of lymph nodes move to the medulla of lymph nodes to secrete antibody.

In secondary responses to TD antigens antibody production characteristically continues for many months. In this situation the response appears to be sustained by B cell activation in association with antigen held on follicular dendritic cells (FDC) [MacLennan et al 1988]. The plasmablasts generated migrate via the lymph and blood to distant sites of antibody production. Where B cells have been activated in the follicles of Peyer's patches or mesenteric lymph nodes the plasmablasts generated migrate to the lamina propria of the gut before becoming plasma cells [Gowans and Knight 1964; Hall et al 1977]. B cells activated in the follicles of the spleen or peripheral lymph nodes become plasma cells in the bone marrow [Benner et al 1981]. Most of these plasma cells produce IgG or IgA antibody. They do not produce IgM. Also the life-span of plasma cells producing IgG or IgA in the rat bone marrow is in the order of 3-4 weeks [Ho et al 1986]. Human bone marrow plasma cells are known to survive in culture, without proliferating for some weeks [Hibi and Dosch 1986].

Some follicular B cell activation is seen in responses to TI-1 antigens. Although these antigens can evoke antibody responses in the absence of T cells it is not clear that the follicular response to TI-2 antigens is T cell independent. Studies of TI-1 antibody responses in euthymic mice and congenic athymic mice have shown that the capacity of these antigens to produce augmented secondary type antibody responses is T cell dependent [Zhang and MacLennan previously unpublished results]. Experiments in rats where TI-2 antigens plus LPS and a TD antigen have been given together show that antibody production to epitopes on the TI-2 antigen can acquire the characteristics of a TD or TI-1 response [Zhang et al 1988b]. These findings make it difficult to extrapolate the site of B cell activation simply by consideration of the specificity of the antibody produced.

THE FOLLICULAR RESPONSE

Although B cell activation in follicles may continue for many months following challenge with a TD antigen the nature of the follicular response varies with time from immunization. During the first month after immunization germinal centers form within follicles. It seems likely that this process is associated with the somatic mutation which occurs in rearranged immunoglobulin genes during TD antibody responses [MacLennan and Gray 1986]. Associated with this process there is a selection mechanism which retains those cells with the highest affinity for antigen on FDC [Liu et al 1989].

Follicular response can be divided conveniently in to three stages [MacLennan et al 1990]. Non-responding (resting) follicles consist of a network of FDC and small recirculating B cells which fill the spaces between the FDC dendritic processes. Following the primary administration of a TD antigen, antibody formation first results from extra-follicular B cell activation [MacLennan et al 1988]. Free antigen then becomes complexed with antibody and is either taken up and catabolized by macrophages or is transported to FDC which retain this for protracted periods [Tew and Mandle 1978, 1979]. Virgin B cells do not appear to have the capacity to respond to antigen pre-localised on FDC [Gray 1988 and MacLennan et al 1990]. It seems likely, however, that a full germinal center response results from the virgin B cells which migrate to follicles following their primary activation in T zones [MacLennan et al 1990]. The number of these primary B blasts which colonize any on follicle is small (less than three) [Kroese et al 1987]. They start to proliferate within the network of the FDC, increasing in numbers exponentially until the spaces in the FDC network become filled with B blasts. At this stage the small recirculating B cells are displaced from the follicle center and form a follicular mantle. The period of growth by the primary follicular B blasts is complete within 3-4 days of the seeding blasts entering the follicles. This marks the end of the first stage of the follicular reaction. As the primary B blasts come to fill the FDC network a dramatic change is triggered in these cells. They appear to leave the center of the FDC network, migrating to one pole of the follicle where they cease to express immunoglobulin on their surface and acquire the characteristic phenotype of centroblasts. Centroblasts, like their progenitors are rapidly proliferating with a cell cycle time of some 6-7 hours [Zhang et al 1988a]. Unlike the primary follicular B blasts, however, they do not increase in numbers for they are continually giving rise to centrocytes. The centrocytes are not in cell cycle and re-express immunoglobulin on their surface. They pass back into the FDC network where many of them die. Evidence from studies of isolated germinal center cells indicate that this results from centrocytes spontaneously entering apoptosis [Liu et al 1989]. This process is prevented if the centrocytes receive a signal through their antigen-specific receptors; a signal, presumably, delivered physiologically by antigen on FDC. This rescue signal does not secure long-term viability of the centrocytes. Additional signals must be delivered if these are to become either memory B cells or migrant plasmablasts. It appears from studies on human tonsil centrocytes that the additional signal inducing memory cell formation is delivered through the surface receptor reacting with CD40 antibodies [Liu et al 1989]. Differentiation to plasmablasts can be secured by the combined exposure to the 25 kDa fragment of the soluble CD23 molecule and IL-1α [Liu, Cairns, Jansen, Bonnefoy, Gordon and MacLennan, previously unpublished observation]. These rescue signals are associated with phenotypic changes in the centrocyte. One of the earliest and most dramatic of these is the expression of the molecule encoded by the <u>bcl</u>-2 oncogene [Liu, Mason, Johnson and MacLennan previously unpublished data].

In the absence of further exposure to free extra-follicular antigen the population of centrocytes gradually declines over a period of some 3 weeks. As the centroblasts die out the supply of centrocytes also dwindles. The loss of the centroblast population marks the end of the second phase of the follicular reaction.

The third and final stage of the follicular response continues throughout the established phase of T cell-dependent antibody responses. This phase is associated with secondary B blasts proliferating in small numbers within follicles; the proliferation being driven by antigen held on FDC. The products of this proliferative activity are memory B cells and migrant plasmablasts. The migrant plasmablasts give rise, depending on the site of the follicular response, to plasma cells in mucosae or the bone marrow. Memory B cells are in equilibrium with the secondary B blasts, in that they are produced by and can give rise to secondary B blasts [MacLennan et al 1990]. On re-challenge with antigen there is compromise between colonization of the FDC network by primary and secondary B blasts so that centroblasts formation is less marked and the FDC network becomes filled, after challenge, in part with secondary B blasts. i.e. the response is a mixture of stages 1 and 2 of the follicular response on the one hand and stage 3 on the other.

THE CHARACTERISTICS OF MIGRANT PLASMABLASTS FROM HUMAN BLOOD AND THEIR POSSIBLE RELATIONSHIP TO THE NEOPLASTIC CELLS IN MYELOMATOSIS

Previously unpublished studies of subsets of human blood B cells have resulted in the isolation and characterization of blood plasmablasts. These cells are included in a fraction of $sCD19^{+}$ $sCD39^{-}sIgD^{-}$ B cells and amount to between a half and one per cent of the blood mononuclear cells of healthy adults.

They have a phenotype (Table) which retains some of the features of germinal center cells in that they express CD77 and to a lesser extent CD38 and CD10. The expression of these molecules by neoplastic cells from some patients with myelomatosis has led to the suggestion that this is a disease

TABLE

The phenotype of migrant plasmablasts, compared to that of their precursors and progeny

B cell subset	In cell cycle?	sCD39	sCD77	sIg	c*bcl*-2	cBU9
Follicular mantle	No	++	-	++	++	-
Centroblasts	Yes	-	++	±	-	-
Centrocyte	No	-	+	+	-	-
Blood Plasmablast	Yes	-	++	+	+	+
Plasma cell	No	+/-	±	-	±	++
RPMI 8266 Myeloma cell line	Yes	-	+	-	+	++

s=surface, c=cytoplasmic, BU9 monoclonal antibody identifying a molecule associated with rough endoplasmic reticulum. The protein encoded by *bcl*-2 was identified by a monoclonal antibody prepared by Dr DY Mason against a peptide based upon the *bcl*-2 gene sequence. This antibody precipitates a 26 kDa protein.

arising in germinal centers [Warburton et al 1989]. The isolation of plasmablasts from normal human blood identifies the possibility that the final event leading to neoplastic transformation in myelomatosis could occur in a cell which has already started to migrate to, or has reached, the bone marrow. Post germinal center features of the migrant plasmablasts from human blood are the expression in their cytoplasm of: the *bcl*-2-encoded protein and the BU9-identified a protein associated with rough endoplasmic reticulum [Ling et al 1987].

The migrant plasmablasts from normal human blood are in cell cycle and have been found to remain in this state with good viability throughout 6-day cultures. The likely transit times for plasmablasts in the blood can be estimated by determining: the number of plasmablasts in the blood; the number of plasma cells in the gut and bone marrow and the life-span of these plasma cells. Taking likely maximum and minimum ranges for these values the transit times for plasmablasts in the blood have been estimated to fall within the range of 1 minute to 8 hours [Chan and MacLennan previously unpublished data]. As this range is less than the likely cell cycle time for migrant plasmablasts, it is unlikely that plasmablasts in the blood are a self renewing population. Physiologically the plasma cells in bone marrow are not in cell cycle [Hibi and Dosch 1986]. Migrant plasmablasts presumably receive a signal causing them to come out of cell cycle at the time they leave the blood to enter the bone marrow stroma. Identification of the this signalling process is clearly relevant to studies of myelomatosis. In many ways the neoplastic cells in this disease resemble plasmablasts which have entered the marrow stroma but have failed, at least in part to come out of cell cycle.

REFERENCES

Benner R, Hijmans W and Haaijman JJ (1981) The bone marrow: the major source of immunoglobulins, but still a neglected site of antibody formation. Clin. Expt. Immunol. **46:** 1

Corbel C. and Melchers F. (1983) Requirement for macrophages or T cell-derived factors in the mitogenic stimulation of murine B cells by LPS. Eur. J. Immunol. **13:** 528

Gowans JL and Knight EJ (1964) The route of recirculation of lymphocytes in the rat. Proc. Roy. Soc.(Lond.) B **159:** 257

Gray D (1988) Recruitment of virgin B cells into an immune response is restricted to activation outside follicles. Immunol. **65:** 73

Hall JG, Hopkins J and Orlans E (1977) Studies on lymphoblasts in the sheep III: The destination of lymph-borne immunoblasts according to their tissue origin. Eur. J. Immunol. **7:** 30

Hibi T and Dosch H-M (1986) Limiting dilution analysis of the B cell compartment of human bone marrow. Eur. J. Immunol. **16:** 139

Ho F, Lortan J, Khan M and MacLennan ICM (1986) Distinct short-lived and long-lived antibody-producing cell populations. Eur. J. Immunol **16:** 1297

Kroese FGM, Wubenna AS, Seijen HG and Nieuwenhuis P (1987) Germinal centers develop oligoclonally. Eur J. Immunol. **17:** 1069

Lane PJL, Gray D and MacLennan ICM (1986) Differences in recruitment of virgin B cells into antibody responses to thymus-dependent and thymus-independent type-2 antigens. Eur. J. Immunol. **16:** 1569

Levit D, Duber-Stull and Lawton RA (1981) T cell-dependent and T cell-independent differentiation induced by E coli lipopolysaccharide in human blood lymphocytes. Clin. Imunol. Immunopathol. **18**: 309

Ling NR, MacLennan ICM and Mason DY (1987) B cell and plasma cell antigens: new and previously defined clusters. p302 in Leukocyte Typing III. eds McMichael et al. Oxford University Press, Oxford.

Leonard RCF, MacLennan ICM, Smart Y, Vanhegan RI and Cuzick J (1979) Light chain isotype-associated suppression of normal plasma cell numbers in patients with multiple myeloma. Int. J. Cancer **24**: 385.

Liu Y-J, Joshua DE, Williams GT, Smith CA, Gordon J and MacLennan ICM (1989) Mechanisms of antigen-driven selection in germinal centres. Nature **342**: 929

MacLennan ICM and Gray D (1986) Antigen-driven selection of virgin and memory B cells. Immunol. rev. **91**: 61

MacLennan ICM, Liu Y-J, Oldfield S, Zhang J and Lane PJL (1990) The Evolution of B cell clones. Current Topics in Microbiol. and Immunol. **159**: 37

MacLennan ICM, Liu Y-J and Ling NR (1988) B cell prololiferation in follicles, germinal centre formation and the site of neoplastic transformation in Burkitt's Lymphoma. Current Topics in Microbiol. Immunol. **141**: 138.

Smith ECI, Hammerstrom L, Bird GA, Kunori T, Gustafson B, and Holm T. (1979) Lipopolysaccharide and lipid A-induced human lymphocyte activation as detected by a protein A plaque assay. Eur. J. Immunol. **9**: 619

Tew JG and Mandel TE (1978) The maintenance and regulation of serum antibody levels: Evidence indicating a role for antigen retained in lymphoid follicles. J. Immunol. **120**: 1063

Tew JG and Mandel TE (1979) Prolonged antigen half-life in the lymphoid follicles of specifically immunized mice. Immunol. **37**: 69

Warburton P, Joshua DE, Gibson J and Brown RD (1989) CD10-(CALLA)-positive lymphocytes in myeloma: evidence that they are a malignant precurssor population and are of germinal centre origin. Leukemia and Lymphoma **1**: 11

Zhang J, MacLennan ICM, Liu Y-J and Lane PJL (1988a) Is rapid proliferation in centroblasts linked to somatic mutation in memory B cell clones? Immunol. Lett. **18**: 297

Zhang J, Liu Y-J, MacLennan ICM, Gray D and Lane PJL (1988b) B cell memory to thymus-independent type 1 and type 2: the role of lipopolysaccharide in B memory induction. Eur. J. Immunol. **18**: 1417

Cytogenetic Abnormalities in Multiple Myeloma

Brian G.M. Durie, Elizabeth E. Vela, Valerie Baum*
Department of Haematology, Charing Cross and Westminster Medical School, University of London, Charing Cross Hospital, Fulham Palace Road London W6
The Arizona Cancer Center, College of Medicine, 1515 North Campbell Avenue, Tucson, Arizona 85724*.

INTRODUCTION

Cytogenic studies in multiple myeloma have been very difficult because of the predominantly low proliferative activity in this disease [1-7]. In the series reported to date the most commonly affected chromosomes have been chromosomes 1 and 14 : a variety of translocations and structural changes have been documented. Chromosome 14 in particular has been involved in translocations to several chromosomes, including t(11;14), t(8;14) and t (14;18) . In addition to these translocations, acquisition of miscellaneous chromosomal fragments and unidentified markers (UMARS) is very frequent. Gains and losses of numerous chromosomes have also been noted. The current report summarises a preliminary analysis of a large study of 331 bone marrow specimens from 262 patients with multiple myeloma, studied at the University of Arizona.

The basic cytogenetic features in the giemsa-banded karyotypes of both treated and untreated patients are reported. Preliminary correlations with patient features and phenotypic and kinetic characteristics of the disease have been conducted.

MATERIALS AND METHODS

Cytogenetic studies were conducted on bone marrow aspirates collected in RPMI 1640 with heparin and colcemid without mitogens (although a variety of potential mitogens were evaluated in parallel studies). Routine methods were used for hypotonic treatment and preparation of air-dried slides[8] . Identical abnormalities in 2 or more cells defined a clonal population except for monosomies or deletions where 3 or more cells with identical aberrations were required[9]. For samples with heterogenous karyotypic changes in different populations, reported karyotypes include all of the clonal abnormalities detected. Normal karyotypes required confirmation of no clonal abnormalities in at least 20 metaphases examined. Detailed phenotypic studies were carried out as previously reported [10-13] (Fig. 1.).

RESULTS

The overall statistics are shown in table 1.

TABLE 1

MYELOMA CYTOGENETICS : OVERALL STATISTICS

		Abnormal Cytogenetics
		Numbers (%)
Total bone marrows studies	331	89/331 (27%)
Total patients studied	262	70/262 (31%)

Patients with abnormal karyotypes	70
Pretreatment	20
Following therapy	50
Serial studies	17

There were 89 abnormal karyotypes in 70 patients. Therefore 70 out of the 262 patients (ie 31%) had abnormal karyotypes. Twenty patients were studied before any treatment had been initiated. Fifty of the 70 patients studied were evaluated during their subsequent course (primarily at relapse), with 17 patients having studies serially during the whole disease course. For comparative purposes detailed karyotypic studies were (Fig. 1.) carried out on 12 established myeloma cell lines (8226, U266, L363, Fravel, Me/CAR, ARH-77 plus 6 LB, lines 83-1, 83-2, 84-1, 84-3, 84-5 and 85-1[8,11]).

Major attention was focused on the cytogenetic abnormalities in the 20 previously untreated patients.

Table 2

COMMON STRUCTURAL ABNORMALITIES IN PREVIOUSLY UNTREATED PATIENTS

Chromosome Number	Break Point
1	p 11-21
	q25
6	q 14-27
7	p 14-22
	q 22-36
14	q32

Eight of these 20 patients had discrete structural abnormalities. The most common breakpoints are listed in table 2 and involved chromosomes number 1, 6 and 7. In addition 3 patients had abnormalities of chromsome 17 and 1 patient with plasma cell leukaemia had a 14q32 abnormality. The identical breakpoints were also noted in > 50% of the 50 previously treated patients, as well as in the 12 established myeloma cell lines (Fig. 1.)

TABLE 3

ADDITIONAL COMMON BREAK POINT ABNORMALITIES IN TREATED PATIENTS AND ESTABLISHED MYELOMA CELL LINES.

Chromosome Number	Breakpoint
14	q+(32 and various)
3	p and q
5	q23-32
11	p15
	q13

However, all of the treated patients and myeloma cell lines had additional cytogenetic abnormalities present. The treated patients and cell lines were more frequently noted to have 14 q+ abnormalities, as well as structural abnormalities of chromosomes 3 p and q, 5q23-32 and 11 p15 and q13. Unidentified markers plus gains and losses of whole chromsomes were extremely common. The predominant gains of chromosomes involved chromosomes 3, 5, 11 and 15. The predominant losses of chromosomes involved, numbers 13, 14, 17 and chromosome x.

TABLE 4

COMMON NUMERIC CHANGES IN PATIENTS WITH ABNORMAL CHROMOSOMES

GAINS	3
	5
	11
	15
LOSSES	13
	14
	17
	X

Seventeen patients had serial cytogenetic studies performed. In each case there were additional chromosomal abnormalities detected in the second and or subsequent samples, as compared to the initial karyotype. There was therefore clear documentation of sequential karyotypic evolution in this subset of patients.

Detailed phenotypic analyses were carried out on the bone marrow myeloma cells from all the patients having karyotypic analysis . Of the 70 patients with abnormal chromosomes, 42 had aberrant myeloma cell phenotypic features. These phenotypic aberrancies included the presence of positive reactions for CALLA [10], myelomonocytic antigens[11,12], T cell antigens[13], as well as p-glycoprotein (C219), using the APAAP cytochemical method (Fig. 1.).

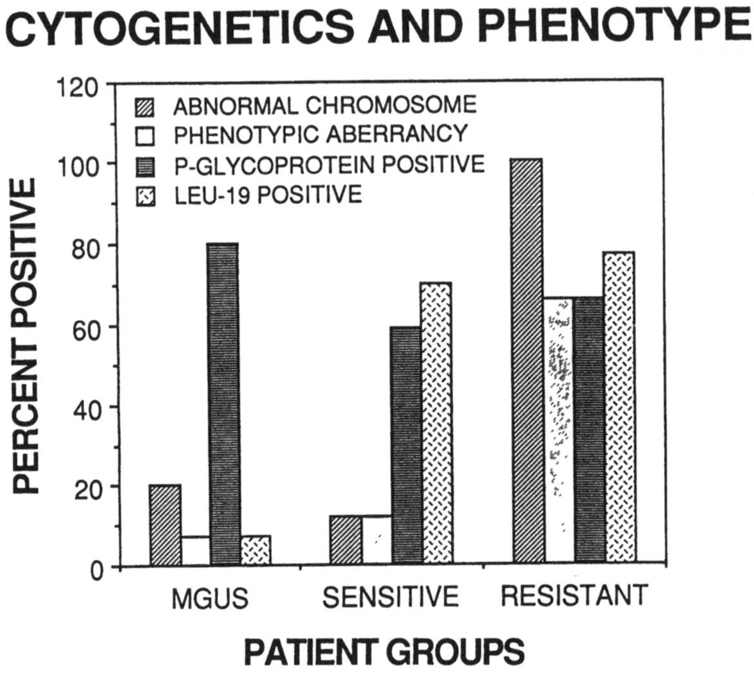

The presence of abnormal chromosomes and also the presence of phenotypic aberrancy predicted for extremely poor overall survival, particularly in patients with relapsing disease who had a median survival of less than 6 months from the point of detection of abnormal chromosomes and/or of phenotypic abnormal changes. The presence of elevated serum beta 2 microglobulin and/or an elevated labelling index also cross correlated with this predicted poor survival. Of interest 3 patients initially diagnosed as having monoclonal gammopathy of undetermined significance (MGUS) had abnormal chromsomes; 2 of these patients subsequently developed multiple myeloma. A very unexpected finding was that patients with MGUS plasma cells were consistently CD56 negative, but were positive in 80% of cases for C219 p-glycoprotein.

DISCUSSION

This preliminary review documents the major structural and numeric abnormalities in a large series of patients with multiple myeloma. The predominant breakpoints in the previously untreated patients, are of particular importance in that they direct attention to areas of special interest. The breakpoints on chromosome 1 (p 11-21) may relate to recently observed mutations in the N-ras oncogene [14]. Breakpoints on chromosome 6q 14-27 may relate to abnormalities of the K-r as or C-MYB oncogenes and numerous important DNA segments may be biologically related to breakpoints on chromosome 7, including V-ERB, IL6, p-glycoprotein and histone. We have previously noted a correlation between 6q chromosome abnormalities and extent of bone disease as well as in vitro OAF production in myeloma patients [15]. Obviously abnormalities on chromosome 14 are closely linked to molecular changes in the immunoglobulin heavy chain gene. Likewise in the treated patients the additional chromsomal changes may have important molecular correlates. More detailed molecular studies are now needed. Detailed studies at both the DNA and RNA levels should prove particularly rewarding in the further evaluation of genetic changes associated with both the pathogenesis of myeloma in untreated patients and the subsequent disease progression with therapy.

REFERENCES

1. Lewis JP, MacKenzie MR (1984): Non-random chromosomal aberrations associated with multiple myeloma. Hematol Oncol 2:307 .
2. DeWald GW, Kyle RA, Hicks GA, Greipp PR (1985): The clinical significance of cytogenetic studies in 100 patients with multiple myeloma, plasma cell leukemia or amyloidosis. Blood 66:380 .
3. Kuey-Chu C, Bevan PC, Mattews JG (1986): Analysis of G banded karyotypes in myeloma cells. J Clin Pathol 39:260.
4. Ranni NS, Slavutsky I, Wechsler A, Brieux S (1987): Chromosome findings in multiple myeloma. Cancer Genet Cytogenet 25:309 .
5. Yamada K, Shionoya S, Amano M, Imamura Y (1983): A Burkitt-type 8;14 translocation in a case of plasma cell leukemia. Cancer Genet Cytogenet 9:67.
6. Nishida K, Taniwaki M, Misawa S, Abe T, Takino T, Fujii H (1987): Translocation (14;18) found in a patient with multiple myeloma. Cancer Genet Cytogenet 25:375.
7. Gould J, Alexanian R, Goodacre A, Pathak S, Hecht B, Barlogie B (1988): Plasma cell karyotype in multiple myeloma. Blood 71:453.8.

8. Durie BGM, Vela E, Baum V, Leibovitz A, Payne CM, Richter LC, Grogan TM, Trent JM (1985): Establishment of two new myeloma cell lines from bilateral pleural effusions: Evidence for sequential in vivo clonal change. Blood 66:548.
9. Harnden GD, Jensen JT (eds) (1985): An international system for human cytogenetic nomenclature. Basel, Switzerland, S. Karges.
10. Durie BGM, Grogan TM (1985): CALLA-positive myeloma: an aggressive subtype with poor survival. Blood 66:229.
11. Durie BGM, Grogan TM, Spier C, Vela E, Baum V, Rodriquez MA, Frutiger Y (1989): Myelomonocytic myeloma cell line (LB 84-1). Blood 73:770.
12. Grogan TM, Durie BGM, Spier CM, Richter L, Vela E (1989): Myelomonocytic antigen positive multiple myeloma. Blood 73:763.
13. Spier C, Durie BGM, Grogan TM, Richter LC, Vela E, Frutiger Y, Rangel CS (May 1990): T cell antigen positive multiple myeloma. Mod Path, in press.
14. Neri A, Murphy JP, Cro L, Ferrero D, Tarella C, Baldini L, Dalla-Favera R (1989): *RAS* oncogene mutation in multiple myeloma. J Exp Med 170:1715.
15. Durie B, Baum V, Vela E, Mundy G (1986): Abnormalities of chromosome 6q and osteoclast activating factor production in multiple myeloma. Blood 68:208A (abstr).

Multiple Myeloma Evolves from a Malignant Hematopoietic Stem Cell

Joshua Epstein and Hiroyuki Hata

Division of Hematology/Oncology, Department of Internal Medicine, University of Arkansas for Medical Science, Arkansas Cancer Research Center, Little Rock, Arkansas 72205.

The low proliferative activity of multiple myeloma cells prompted investigations designed to identify the proliferative pool of pre-myeloma cells which feed into the compartment of recognizable tumor cells. In the last several years significant insight has been gained into the biology of myeloma; the involvement of pre-B lymphocytes has been demonstrated, IL-6 has been identified as the major myeloma growth factor, the role of accessory cells has been recognized and the efficacy of biologicals with known activity as regulators of gene expression in controlling the disease has been established. Yet the myeloma stem cell has remained elusive.

In the absence of a myeloma-specific genetic lesion which would allow recognition of normal-appearing involved cells, elaborate indirect approaches have to be taken to gain insight into the ontogeny of myeloma. Recent findings from several laboratories may provide guiding clues in the search of the myeloma stem cells.

The first genetic event during commitment to B-cell differentiation is rearrangement of the immunoglobulin (Ig) heavy chain genes. This is followed by rearrangements of the light chain Kappa gene followed by Lambda. Clonal rearrangements in the Ig genes are proof to the clonality of myeloma as well as the other B-cell malignancies, and are frequently analyzed in the diagnostic and research laboratories. Occasionally, rearrangements in heavy or light chain gene only are detected, even in samples containing considerable proportions of myeloma cells with unequivocal production and secretion of immunoglobulins. The bone marrow sample from patient H. had 65% aneuploid myeloma cells containing both Kappa and Lambda light chain cytoplasmic immunoglobulins. When analyzed for Ig gene rearrangements, J_H and Kappa genes had a rearranged allele but only germline Lambda gene was seen. Patient D., also expressing Kappa and Lambda cIg, had rearranged J_H but only germline Kappa. Both patients had M protein of the IgG/Lambda type. Such findings are not uncommon among investigators and often solicit apologetic explanations or mere acknowledgement. Yet germline Ig gene expression has been described (Nelson, Kelley and Perry 1985, Schlissel and Baltimore 1989). It likely occurs normally, although perhaps in a low frequency, during B-cell differentiation. However, if occurring in a malignant, pre-myeloma cell immortalized by neoplastic transformation, the result following expansion would be a germline Ig gene expressing myeloma. It is also possible that such anomalies are more likely to occur in neoplastically transformed cells, albeit in low frequency. This too would imply that myeloma arises from a cell which is already transformed when it reaches the differentiation stage of Ig gene rearrangement.

Patient H also had rearranged T cell receptor (TcR)-δ and -τ genes, and patient D had a rearranged TcR-δ gene (Table 1). Rearranged TcR-τ and TcR-δ genes have been reported also in other B-cell neoplasms (Greaves et.al. 1986, Lee et.al. 1987, Dyer 1989).

TABLE 1.

PATIENT	M-PROTEIN	cIg	J_H	KAPPA	LAMBDA	TcR-δ	TcR-τ
H	IgG-Lambda	K+L	R/G[a]	R/G	G/G	R/G	R/G
D	IgG-Lambda	K+L	R/G	G/G	G/G	R/G	G/G

[a] R: Rearranged allele; G: Germline

TcR gene rearrangements are the initial genetic events in commitment to differentiation along the T lymphocyte lineage, in parallel to the Ig gene rearrangements in commitment to B-cell differentiation. Infidelity in these events is likely to occur normally in low frequency, resulting in non-functional and non-viable cells. If occurring in a transformed pre-tumor cell, this infidelity will be detected eventually in the neoplastic cell population. This could be interpreted to suggest that an early lymphoid cell, at a differentiation stage prior to T- and B-cell commitment, is involved in myeloma, and indeed in the other B-cell neoplasias.

Analysis of expression of lineage- and differentiation-associated surface molecules is a powerful tool in the diagnosis of immune system disorders and in the classification of neoplastic diseases of the hematopoietic system. Such analyses led to the demonstration of B-cell involvement in myeloma and to the delineation of a pre-myeloma compartment at a maturation level of pre-B cells (Grogan et.al. 1987, Epstein et.al. 1988). Expression of several lineage-restricted antigens by leukemic cells from patients with acute myeloid leukemia suggested multilineage involvement (Keinänen et.al. 1988). Expression of myeloid antigens by myeloma cells, reported byGrogan et.al. (1989), is reminiscent of the mixed leukemias in which tumor cells express both myeloid and lymphoid antigens, and suggests the involvement of the myeloid cell lineage in myeloma. More recently it was reported that myeloma cells frequently express megakaryocytic, erythroid and myelomonocytic genes together with typical myeloma-associated features (Epstein, Xiao and He 1990).

Multilineage marker expression (also termed "lineage infidelity") such as has been described in AML, the mixed leukemias and more recently in multiple myeloma, could be explained by the loss of regulatory control in malignant cells. Expression of multilineage genes would represent "de-differentiation", where the malignant cells express genes which were never expressed or which were turned off several differentiation steps prior to the transformation event. The apparent pattern in the repertoire of aberrantly expressed genes (e.g. 88% of myeloma patients expressing megakaryocytic markers while only 39% with erythroid marker expression) could be explained by the relative "leakiness" of these genes. However, this explanation can not be applied to the genetic evidence of lineage "infidelity" such as clonal TcR gene rearrangements in B-cell tumors.

A second scenario, more compatible with the available data, would have the initial malignant lesion in a pluripotential hematopoietic stem cell. As this cell progresses along the differentiation pathway, genetic events associated with the process are regulated with a lesser than normal degree of stringency. The resulting multilineage marker expression would not represent "de-differentiation" but rather uncontrolled progression through the differentiation process. This not only suggests that myeloma originates from a malignant hematopoietic stem cell, but also that all malignant diseases of the hematopoietic system originate from a malignant hematopoietic stem cell. Secondary tumor promotion events, possibly in association with specific cell lineage turn-over rates, determine the phenotypic expression of the tumor.

REFERENCES

Dyer MJ (1989) T-cell receptor δ/α rearrangements in lymphoid neoplasms. Blood 74:1073-1083.

Epstein J, Barlogie B, Katzmann F, Alexanian R (1988) Phenotypic heterogeneity in aneuploid multiple myeloma indicates pre-B cell involvement. Blood 71:861-865.

Epstein J, Xiao H, He XY (1990) Markers of multiple hematopoietic-cell lineage in multiple myeloma. N Engl J Med 322:664-668.

Greaves MF, Chan LC, Furley AJW, Watt SM, Molgaard HV (1986) Lineage promiscuity in hematopoietic differentiation and leukemia. Blood 76:1-11.

Grogan TM, Durie BG, Lomen C, Spier C, Wirt DP, Nagle R, Wilson GS, Richter L, Vela E, Maxey V, McDaniel K, Rangel C (1987) Delineation of a novel pre-B component in plasma cell myeloma: Immunochemical, immunophenotypic, genotypic, cytologic, cell culture and kinetic features. Blood 70:932-942.

Grogan TM, Durie BG, Spier CM, Richter L, Vela E (1989) Myelomonocytic antigen positive multiple myeloma. Blood 73:763-769.

Keinänen M, Griffin JD, Bloomfield CD, Machnicki J, de la Chapelle A (1988) Clonal chromosomal abnormalities showing multiple-cell-lineage involvement in acute myeloid leukemia. N Engl J Med 318:1153-1158.

Lee M, Selvanayagam P, Alexanian R, Stass S, Barlogie B (1987) Rearrangement (REARR) of T-cell receptor (TcR) γ chain gene in multiple myeloma (MM). Proc Am Assoc Cancer Res 28:178.

Nelson KJ, Kelley DE, Perry RP (1985) Inducible transcription of the unrearranged K constant region locus is a common feature of pre-B cells and does not require DNA or protein synthesis. Proc Natl Acad Sci USA 82:5305-5309.

Schlissel MS, Baltimore D (1989) Activation of immunoglobulin kappa gene rearrangement correlates with induction of germline gene transcription. Cell 58:1001-1007.

Amylase-Producing Multiple Myeloma

H. Matsuzaki, H. Hata, I. Sanada*, and K. Takatsuki

The Second Department of Internal Medicine, Kumamoto University Medical School, Honjo 1-1-1, Kumamoto 860, Japan.
*The Department of Internal Medicine, Kumamoto National Hospital, Ninomaru 1-5, Kumamoto 860, Japan.

INTRODUCTION

Hyperamylasemia resulting from ectopic production of amylase by tumor tissue was first described by Weiss et al.(1951). Since then, several cancer cases of hyperamylasemia have been reported, including lung (Maeda et al. 1982; Katayama et al. 1981; Braganza et al. 1978; Yokoyama et al. 1977), ovary (Hodes et al. 1985; Cramer et al. 1979; Sandiford et al. 1978; Corlette et al. 1978), stomach (Nomura et al. 1980), and others (Yoshimura et al. 1986; Ueda et al. 1977; Matsuyama et al. 1979; Weitzel et al. 1988; Maesiar 1984). Most of these have been derived from epithelial tissues. To our knowledge, we reported the first case of an amylase-producing multiple myeloma (Hata et al. 1988). We also established an amylase-producing multiple myeloma cell line, KHM-1B from the patient (Matsuzaki et al. 1988).

Although a number of amylase-producing tumors have been identified, the mechanism of amylase production by tumor cell is not well understood. KHM-1B are useful tool for analysis of ectopic amylase production. In order to understand the mechanism of ectopic amylse production, we analyzed the karyotype, DNA and RNA of the KHM-1B(Hata et al. in press).

MATERIALS AND METHODS

Case Report

The patient was a 53-year-old man first admitted to the hospital in May 1985 for epigastralgia. A gastric ulcer and hyperamylasemia were identified, and a wide gastrectomy was done one month later because perforation of the ulcer to the pancreas was suspected as a cause of the continued hyperamylasemia. However, no lesion was found in the pancreas, and the cause of the hyperamylasemia was not found. The hyperamylasemia persisted after the operation, and 6 months later, the patient complained of pain in the right upper arm. Radiologic examination revealed a punched-out lesion of the right humerus, the biopsy specimen of which showed a plasmacytoma. For this reason he was transferred to our hospital.

On admission he had hemoglobin of 11.5g/dl, leukocyte of 11,500/mm^3, with 2% plasma cells, and erythrocytes of 3,720x10^3/mm^3. Bone marrow aspiration revealed a nuclear cell count of 164x10^3/mm^3, with 36.5% plasma cells. Bence Jones protein was found in his urine. Laboratory data were as follows: total protein 9.8g/dl ($\beta + \gamma$ 49.3%, consisting of IgA-λ type M-protein); IgG, 793mg/dl; IgA, 3,804mg/dl; IgM, 35mg/dl; and amylase, 1,600U/L (S-type activity determined by amylase inhibitor method was 90%). Radiologic examination revealed multiple punched-out lesions on many bones, including the skull and femur. Hyperamylasemia and high serum IgA levels were improved by treatment with melphalan and prednisolone (Fig.1).

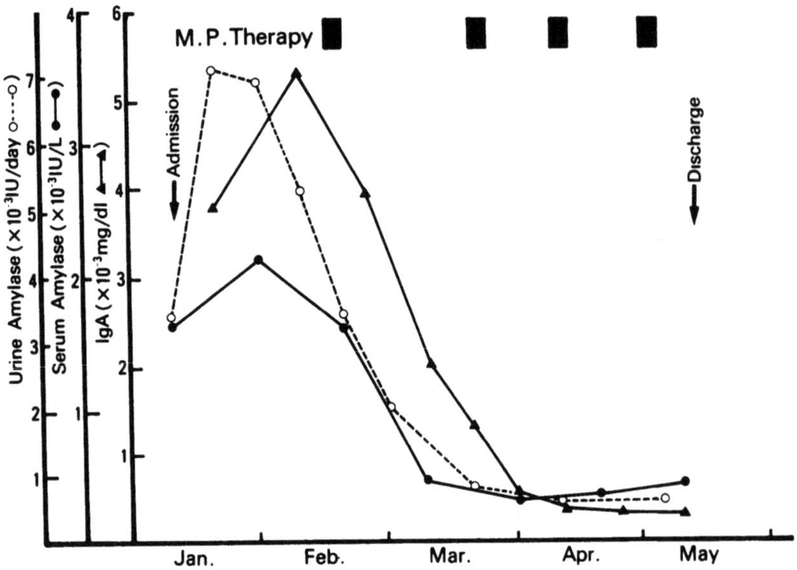

Fig. 1. Levels of amylase activity in the urine and serum and IgA levels in the serum during hospitalization. Rapid decreases in both IgA and amylase levels were obeserved during chemotherapy.
○---○ : Urine amylase; ●—● : Serum amylase; ▲—▲ : IgA.

Although the patient was discharged in improved condition in May 1986, he was readmitted in August 1986 because of a plasmacytoma in the left chest wall. Despite intensive chemotherapy with cyclophosphamide, vindesine, doxorubicin, and prednisolone, he developed malignant pleural effusion from plasma cells, right femoral fracture, and hypercalcemia. He died of pneumonia in November 1986. Post-mortem examination detected no primary lesions in either the pancreas or the salivary glands. Plasmacytomas were found in the left chest wall, retroperitoneum, and liver (Takeya et al. 1989).

Cell Culture

Heparinized pleural effusions from the patient were layered on the Ficoll-Conray (specific gravity, 1.078) and were centrifuged at 400g for 30 minutes. The interphase cells, which consisted almost entirely of myeloma cells, were collected and seeded into culture plates at approximately 10^6 cells/ml after washing with complete medium. In primary culture and the early passages, RPMI 1640 medium containig 20% fetal calf serum (FCS) was used, but when the cells began to grow steadily, the medium was changed to RPMI 1640 containing 10% FCS. The cells were maintained throughout under 5% CO_2 in humidified air at 37°C.

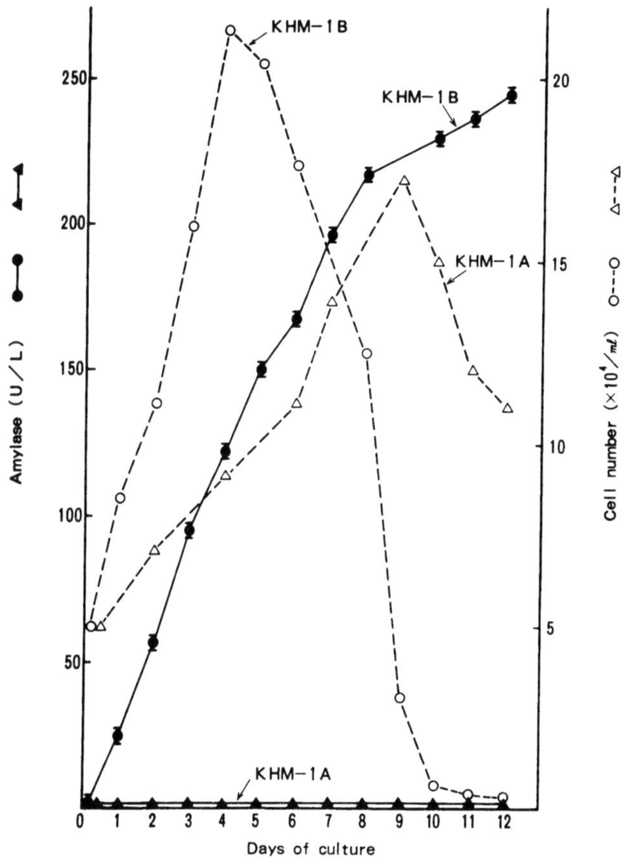

Fig. 2. Cell number and amylase secretion. Cell number (○ , △) and amylase activity (● , ▲) in the culture medium were assayed daily for 12 days. No medium changes were made during the experiment.

Southern Blot Analysis

DNA was analyzed as described previously (Southern 1975). Briefly, 10 µg of high molecular weight DNA was digested with the appropriate restriction enzymes, electrophoresed in 0.7% agarose gel and transferred to a nitrocellulose filter. After being prehybridized at 42°C in 5 X standard saline citrate (SSC), 5 X Denhart's solution, 50% formamide, 20nM sodium phosphate buffer and heat denatured salmon sperm DNA (200 µg/ml), filters were hybridized with ^{32}P-labeled c-DNA probe at 42°C, wased three times at room temperature with 5 X SSC/0.1% sodium dodecyl sulfate (SDS) and then washed again at 56°C with 0.1 X SSC/0.1% SDS. Finally, filters were exposed to X-ray with intensifying screeens overnight at -70°C.

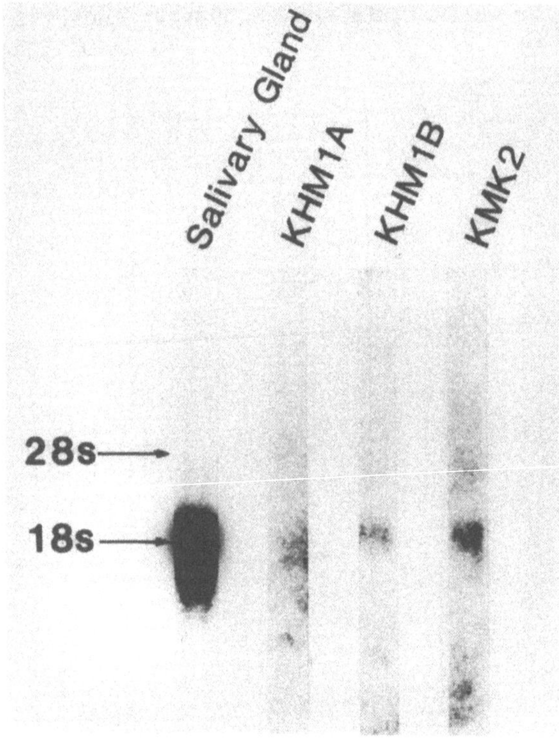

Fig. 3. Expression of amylase m-RNA in a normal salivary gland, KHM-1B and KMK-2 cells. The total m-RNA used from the salivary gland and amylase-producing cell lines was 2 and 20 µg, respectively. m-RNA were electorophoresed in 1% agarose gel containing 2.2M formaldehyde, transferred to a nitrocellulose filter, and hybridized with ^{32}P-labeled amylase c-DNA probe as described in materials and methods.

Northern Blot Analysis

Total cellular RNA was extracted from cells using the guanidine thiocyanate/cesium chloride method as described elsewhere (Chirgwin et al. 1979). A normal human salivary gland was frozen in liquid nitrogen, cut into small pieces with a Waring Blender (New Hartford, Conneticut) and used as the source of RNA. 10 µg of total RNA was denatured by heating at 60°C for 20 minutes in 50% (vol/vol) formamide and electrophoresed in 1% agarose gel containing 2.2 M formaldehyde. After transferring the RNA to nitrocellulose filters, the filters were baked for 2 hours at 80°C followed by hybridization, washing and autoradiography as in Southern blotting. c-DNA probe, a 1.62 kb Pst1-Pst1 fragment containing human P-type amylase gene (Nakamura et al. 1984) was kindly provided by Prof.

Matsubara of the Institute of Cellular and Molecular Biology, Osaka University.

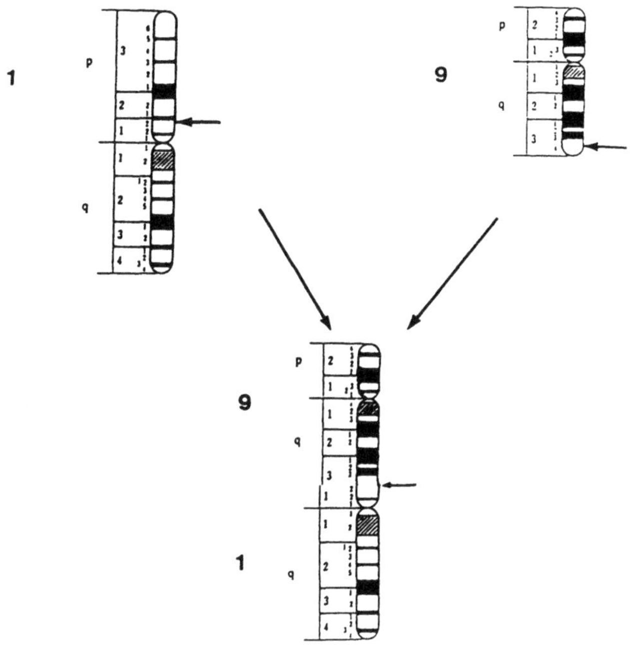

Fig. 4. Scheme of t(1;9)(p13-21;q34) recognized in KHM-1B. Arrows indicate break-points.

RESULTS

Establishment of Amylase Producing Myeloma Cell Line

The myeloma cells were collected and cultured from the patient's pleural effusions. At early passage, the two types of cells obtained, called KHM-1A and KHM-1B, floated in the culture medium almost as single-cell suspensions. At a later passage, however, their characteristics gradually diverged. KHM-1A cells tended to attach singly to the plastic substratum, whreas KHM-1B cells formed soft clusters that continued to float. In Wright-Giemasa-stained smears, both KHM-1A and KHM-1B cells were morphologically similar to typical plasmablasts, having nuclei containing necleoli and basophilic cytoplasm. Immunoperoxidase studies using anti-amylase antibody showed that most KHM-1B cells were positive, whereas practically no KHM-1A cells were positive.

Both KHM-1A and KHM-1B cells were positive for HLA-DR and PCA-1 but negative for CD 2 (OKT 11), CD 10 (CALLA), and CD 20 (Leu 16). Living cells were analyzed with the fluorescein-conjugated anti-immunoglobulin antisera for sIgs and were found to be unstainable.

With fixed cells, α chain and λ immunoglobulins were detected in the cytoplasm.

Cell numbers and amylase activities of culture medium were assayed serially without medium changes to determine the accumulation with time of amylase in the culture medium. The doubling time of KHM-1A cells was about five days and that of KHM-1B was about two days (Fig.2). An almost linear increase in amylase activity in the culture medium of KHM-1B cells was observed until day 12 of cultivation, but no amylase activity was detected in the culture medium of KHM-1A cells (fig.2).

Genetic Analysis of Amylase Producing Myeloma Cell Line

Northern blot analysis showed production of S-type amylase at the m-RNA level by KHM-1B but KHM-1A (Fig.3). Normal salivary gland and KMK-2 which is an S-type amylase producing gastric cancer cell line, were used as positive controls.

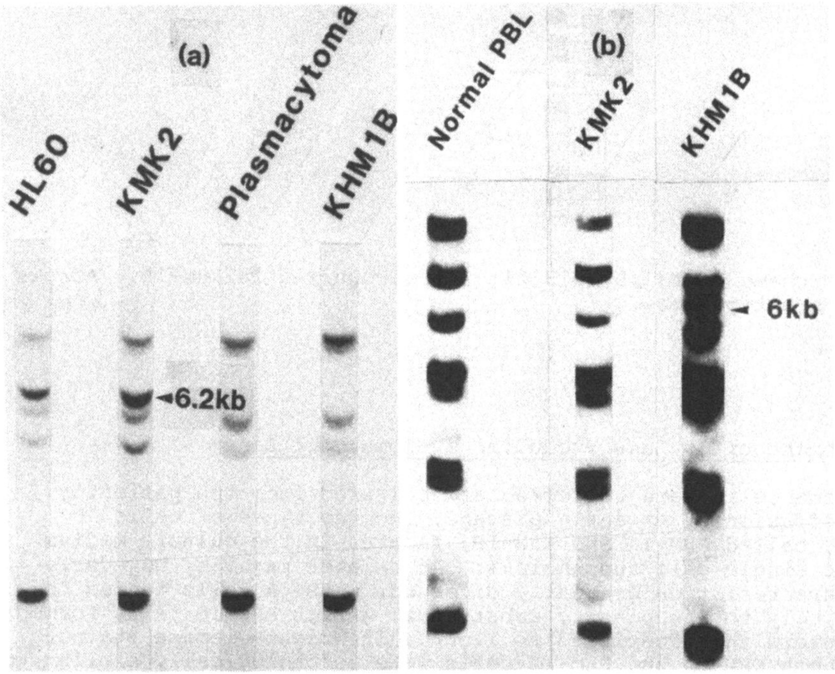

Fig. 5. Southern blot analysis of KHM-1B after Acc1 digestion. Cla1-Pst1 (a) and Bgl2-EcoR1 (b) fragment of P-type amylase cDNA were used as probes. High molecular weight DNA was digested with Acc1, electrophoresed in 0.7% agarose gel, transferred to nitrocellulose filter, and hybridized with ^{32}P-labeled amylase c-DNA probe as described in materials and methods. Deletion of the 6.2kb band (A) and appearance of a 6kb (B) were observed.

Karyotypic analysis revealed many abnormalities in KHM-1B cells (Hata et al. in press). The most interesting finding in the cell line was the translocation observed between 1p13 or 21, near the locus of the amylase gene, and 9q34, the locus of the abl oncogene (Fig.4). On the other hand, the karyotype of KMK-2 showed no traslocation involving the amylase gene.

In Southern blot analysis, KMK-2 revealed no abnormalities. As for KHM-1B, a rearranged band was observed in the case of digestion by Accl. Disappearance of the 6.2kb band and appearance of a 6.0kb band were observed when P-amylase Cla1-Pst1 probe and Bgl2-EcoR1 fragment were used as probes (Fig.5). No rearrangement of the v-abl gene was found in KHM-1B. Because the same genetic abnormality was detected in KHM-1A, amylase production by KHM-1A and KHM-1B may be not qualitative but quantitative difference.

DISCUSSION

Malignant plasma cells have proved to be very difficult to establish, and only a limited number of human myeloma cell lines have been reported (Matsuoka et al. 1967; Nilsson et al. 1970; Jobin et al. 1974; Burk et al. 1978; Karpas et al. 1982; Miller et al. 1982; Togawa et al. 1982; Niho et al. 1984; Durie et al. 1985; Gazdar et al. 1986; Ohtsuki et al. 1989). We established two EBV-negative subclonal myeloma cell lines. Routine light microscopy, immunohistochemistry, and electron microscopy indicated that they had plasma cell morphologies that were retained in long-term culture. Production and secretion of monoclonal IgA λ immunoglobulin, the same serum isotype as the patient's monoclonal protein, by both myeloma cell lines was observed by immunoperoxidase staining, PFC assay, and ELISA (Matsuzaki et al. 1988). In addition, KHM-1B cells were found to produce and secrete α-amylase. As already mentioned, many cases of ectopic amylase production by tumors have been reported, especially in pulmonary and ovarian cancers, but to our knowledge, this was the first case of an amylase-producing hematopoietic cancer. In addition, KHM-1B was only the second reported amylase-producing cell line. The first amylase-producing cell line, KMK-2, was established from the patient with gastric cancer by Nomura et al. (1980) at Kumamoto University Medical School.

The production of various hormones by cancer cells has been recognized and interpreted as an ectopic phenotype. Amylase produced by cancer cells may represent another example of an ectopically produced enzyme. However, the mechanism of amylase production from tumor cells is not well understood. Several theories have been presented in regard to this mechanism. First, amylase could be overproduced in tumors which normally synthesize amylase, e.g., lung (Otsuki et al. 1977), liver (Arnold et al. 1963) and oviduct (Hochberg 1974). In fact, most cancer patients with hyperamylasemia have pulmonary or ovarian cancers. Tomita et al. (1988) demonstrated the presence of amylase m-RNA in 15 out of 17 cases of lung adenocarcinoma and speculated that lung adenocarcinoma may have originated from cells which are normally or potentially capable of producing amylase. A second possibility is that the amylase gene is activated by unknown mechanism associated with oncogenesis.

It is possible that a chromosomal translocation results in amylase gene activation similar to myc and bcl-2 oncogene activation in Burkitt lymphoma with t(8;14) (Dunnick et al. 1983) and follicular lymphoma with t(14;18) (Cossman et al. 1985). The translocaiton obseved between 1p13 or 21 and 9q34 in the KHM-1B cell line enables us to speculate that there could be a close relationship between the translocation and activation of the amylase gene. That is, the amylase locus at 1p21, may have been translocated to an upstream enhancer gene or oncogene. Although it was not proven that the abl oncogene at 9q34 affects the amylase gene in this way, abl oncogene may lead to the activation of the amylase gene. Because abnormal bands were observed only in the case of digestion of KHM-1B by Accl, the shifted band may be the result of polymorphism. However, according to the genomic restriction map of the amylase gene analyzed by Nishide et al. (1986), there is no explanation for such abnormal bands. Moreover, DNA obtained from 10 healthy donors revealed no abnormal bands in the case of Accl digestion.

KMK-2 showed no amylase gene translocation in karyotypic analysis and no shifted bands were revealed by Southern blot analysis. Epithelial amylase-producing tumors, such as KMK-2, may be subject to a different mechanism of amylase gene activation from than KHM-1B, a non-epithelial tumor. Investigation of the similarities and differences between the amylase-producing mechanisms of these two cell lines has provided important information. Further analysis of these cell lines, utilizing other approaches such as pulse field electrophoresis and genomic sequence analysis of 3' side of the amylase gene, is required.

Since we reported the first case of amylase-producing myeloma, eight other cases have been successively reported in the Japanese literature (Hata et al. 1988; Matsuzaki et al. 1988, 1989; Ohtsuki et al. 1989; Yamazaki et al. 1990; Yagata et al. 1979; Kanno et al. 1988). Two other amylase-producing myeloma cell lines were also established. Karyotypic analysis of two cell lines indicated the chromosome abnormalities on near the region of amylase gene, 1p21. One was del(1)(p22-pter) (Ohtsuki et al. 1988), and the other was t(1;8;14)(p21,2; q24,1; q32,3) (Proceedings of the 31th Annual Meeting of the Japan Clinical Hematological Society 30: 1562, 1989). We are now seeking information on amylase-producing myeloma from abroad. Karyotype analysis of many other cases is important to understand the mechaniam of ectopic production by myeloma cells.

SUMMARY

A patient with IgA lambda type multiple myeloma who appeared to be secreting salivary type amylase ectopically is reported. An amylase producing cell line, KHM-1B was established from the patient. Chromosome analysis of KHM-1B showed many qualitative and quantitative abnormalities including a translocation between 1p13 or 21, near the amylase gene locus, and 9q34, the abl oncogene locus. These finding suggest that the amylase gene in KHM-1B is activated by the translocation. A rearranged amylase gene was demonstrated by Southern blot analysis with only one enzyme, Accl.

REFERENCES

Arnold M, Rutter WJ (1963) Liver amylase III. Synthesis by the perfused liver and secretion into the perfusion medium. J Biol Chem 238: 2760-2765

Braganza JM, Butler EB, Fox H, Hunter PM, Qureshi MSA, Samarji W, Vallon AG (1978) Ectopic producion of salivary type amylase by a pseudomesotheliomatous carcinoma of the lung. Cancer 41: 1522-1525
Burk KH, Drewinko B, Trujollo JM, Ahearn MJ (1978) Establishment of a human plasma cell line in vitro. Cancer Res 38: 2508-2513
Chirgwin J, Przybla H, MacDonald R, Rutter W (1979) Isolation of biologically active ribonucleic acid from sources enriched in ribonuclease. Biochem 18: 5294-5299
Corlette MB, Dratch M, Sorger K (1978) Amylase elevation attributable to an ovarian neoplasm. Gastroenterology 74: 907-909
Cossman J, Jaffe E, Croce CM (1985) Involvement of the bcl-2 gene in human follicular lymphoma. Science 228: 1440-1443
Cramer SF, Bruns DE (1979) Amylase-producing ovarian neoplasm with pseudo-Meigs' syndrome and elevated pleural fluid amylase. Cancer 44: 1715-1721
Dunnick W, Shell BE, Dery C (1983) DNA sequences near the site of reciprocal recombination between a c-myc oncogene and immunoglobulin switch region. Proc Natl Acad Sci USA 80: 7269-7273
Durie BGM, Vela E, Baum V, Leibovitz A, Payne CM, Richter LC, Grogan TM, Trent JM (1985) Establishment of two new myeloma cell lines from bilateral pleural effusions: Evidence for sequential in vivo clonal change. Blood 66: 548-555
Gazdar AF, Oie HK, Kirsch IR, Hollis GF (1986) Establishment and characterization of a human plasma cell myeloma culture having a rearranged cellular myc proto-oncogene. Blood 67: 1542-1549
Hata H, Matsuzaki H, Tanaka K, Nomura H, Kagimoto T, Takeya M, Yamane N, Takatsuki K (1988) Ectopic producion of salivary-type amylase by a IgA-λ-type multiple myeloma. Cancer 62: 1511-1515
Hata H, Matsuzaki H, Sanada I, Takatsuki K (in press) Genetic analysis of amylase-producing cell lines: Ectopic activation of the amylase gene by translocation. Jpn J Clin Oncol in press
Hochberg CJ (1974) Tubal amylase. Obstet Gynecol 43: 129-131
Hodes ME, Sisk CJ, Karn RC, Ehrlich CE, Lehrner LM, Roth LM, Morley DJ, Merritt AD (1985) An amylase-producing serous cystadenocarcinoma of the ovary. Oncology 42: 242-247
Jobin ME, Fahey JL, Price Z (1974) Long-term establishment of a human plasmacyte cell line derived from a patient with IgD multiple myeloma. I. Requirement of a plasmacyte-stimulating factor for proliferation of myeloma cells in tissue culture. J Exp Med 140: 494-507
Kanno M, Ohtake S, Okafuji K, Hirai J, Itoh K, Kobayashi K, Yoshida T, Nakamura S, Matsuda T (1988) IgD-type multiple myeloma associated with tumor of the pancreas. Jpn J Clin Hematol 29: 2312-2316
Karpas A, Ficher P, Swirsky D (1982) Human palsmacytoma with an unusual karyotype growing in vitro and producing light-chain immunoglobulin. Lancet April 24: 931-933
Katayama S, Ikeuchi M, Kanazawa Y, Akanuma Y, Kosaka K, Takeuchi T, Nakayama T (1981) Amylase-producing lung cancer. Cancer 48: 2499-2502
Maeda M, Otsuki M, Yuu H, Saeki S, Yamasaki T, Baba S (1982) Salivary-type hyperamylasemia in primary lung cancer. Eur J Cancer Clin Oncol 18: 123-128
Maesiar PJ (1984) Serum amylase and isoamylase in malignant bone tumors. Neoplasma 31: 351-359
Matsuoka Y, Moore GE, Yagi Y, Pressman D (1967) Production of free light chains of immunoglobulin by a hematopoietic cell line

derived from a patient with multiple myeloma. Proc Soc Exp Biol Med 125: 1246-1250
Matsuyama M, Inoue T, Ariyoshi Y, Doi M, Suchi T, Sato T, Tashiro K, Chihara T (1979) Argyrophil cell carcinoma of the cervix with ectopic production of ACTH, ß-MSH, serotonin, histamin and amylase. Cancer 44: 1813-1823
Matsuzaki H, Hata H, Takeya M, Takatsuki K (1988) Establishment and characterization of an amylse-producing human myeloma cell line. Blood 72: 978-982
Matsuzaki H, Takatsuki K (1989) Amylase producing multiple myeloma. Blood 74: 889
Miller CH, Carbonell A, Peng R, Paglieroni T, MacKenzie MR (1982) A human plasma cell line. Induction and characterization. Cancer 49: 2091-2096
Nakamura Y, Ogawa M, Nishide T, Emi M, Kosaki G, Himeno S, Matubara K (1984) Sequences of cDNAs for human salivary and pancreatic alpha-amylases. Gene 28: 263-270
Niho Y, Shibuya T, Yamasaki K, Kimura N (1984) The establishment of a human myeloma cell line elaborating λ-light chain protein. Int J Cell Cloning 2: 161-172
Nilsson K, Bennich H, Johansson SGO, Ponten J (1970) Established immunoglobulin producing myeloma (IgE) and lymphoblastoid (IgG) cell lines from an IgE myeloma patient. Clin Exp Immunol 7: 477-489
Nishide T, Nakamura Y, Emi M, Yamamoto T, Ogawa M, Mori T, Matsubara K (1986) Primary structure of human salivary alpha-amylase gene. Gene 41: 299-304
Nomura H, Tokumitsu S, Takeuchi T (1980) Ultrastructual, cytochemical, and biochemical characterization of alpha-amylase produced by human gastric cancer cells in vitro. JNCI 64: 1015-1020
Ohtsuki T, Yawata Y, Wada H, Sugihara T, Mori M, Namba M (1989) Two human myeloma cell lines, amylase-producing KMS-12-PE and amylase-non-producing KMS-12-BM, were established from a patient, having the same chromosome marker, t(11;14)(q13;q32). Br J Haematol 72: 199-204
Otuki M, Yuu H, Maeda M, Saeki S, Yamasaki T, Baba S (1977) Amylase in the lung. Cancer 39: 1656-1663
Sandiford JA, Chiknas SG (1979) Hyperamylasemia and ovarian carcinoma. Clin Chem 25: 948-950
Southern EM (1975) Detection of Specific sequences among DNA fragment separated by gel electrophoresis. J Mol Biol 98: 503-517
Takeya M, Matsuzaki H, Hata H, Takatsuki K, Takahashi K (1989) Amylase-producing multiple myeloma: Cytochemical, immunohistochemical and immunoelectron microscopic studies. Virchows Archiv A Pathol Anat 415: 219-224
Togawa A, Inoue N, Miyamoto K, Hyodo H, Namba M (1982) Establishment and characterization of a human myeloma cell line (KMM-1). Int J Cancer 29: 495-500
Tomita N, Matsuura N, Horii A, Emi M, Nishide T, Ogawa M, Mori T, Doi O, Matsubara K (1988) Expression of α-amylase in human lung cancers. Cancer Res 48: 3292-3296
Ueda M, Kobayashi M, Taketa K, Sato J (1977) Ectopic production of a salivary type amylase by adenocarcinoma cells: Demonstration by a culture technique. Clin Chim Acta 80: 105-111
Weiss MJ, Edmondson HA, Wertman M (1951) Elevated serum amylase associated with bronchogenic carcinoma. Report of a case. Am J Clin Pathol 21: 1057-1061
Weitzel JN, Pooler PA, Mohammed R, Levitt MD Eckfeldt JH (1988) A

unique case of breast carcinoma producing pancreatic-type isoamylase. Gastroenterol 94: 519-520
Yagata M (1979) Isozyme of amylase. Lab Friends 10: 3-14 (in Japanese)
Yamazaki T, Matsuura S, Watanabe K, Osato M, Waku S, Saito K, Enokihara H, Furusawa S, Shishido H (1990) Amylase-producing extramedullary plasmacytoma with multiple cutaneous metastasis following a solitary plasmacytoma of bone. Jpn J Clin Hematol 31: 391-395
Yokoyama M, Natsuizaka T, Ishii Y, Ohshima S, Kasagi A, Tateno S (1977) Amylase-producing lung cancer. Cancer 40: 766-772
Yoshimura Y, Oka M, Sugihara T, Mishima K (1986) Lymphoepithelial (brachial) cyst and amylase. Int J Oral Maxillofac Surg 15: 196-200

Experimental Studies

The C57BL/KaLwRij Mouse Model of B-Cell Proliferative Disorders. Is there a Relationship Between Benign Monoclonal Gammopathy and Multiple Myeloma ?

J. Radl

TNO Institute for Experimental Gerontology, Rijswijk, The Netherlands

The C57BL/KaLwRij mice have been shown to spontaneously develop a variety of B-cell proliferative disorders with aging. Over 80% of mice of this strain develop benign monoclonal gammopathy (BMG) which in most aspects is indistinguishable from that described in humans (for reviews see Radl,1981, 1986, 1989). About one third of old mice at necropsy and histopathology examination were shown to suffer from lymphoma, mainly of the follicle center cell type, the majority of which is most likely of the B cell origin (unpublished results). Nearly 1% of mice older than two years develop Waldenström's macroglobulinaemia-like lymophoma (WM) (Radl et al. 1989) or multiple myeloma (MM) (Radl et al. 1988). So far, only BMG and MM have been studied in more detail. Results of these studies can briefly be summarized as follows:

BMG

BMG is a monoclonal proliferative disorder characterized by a non-progressive expansion of an Ig-producing clone, which resides mainly in the bone marrow in a diffuse pattern. The clonal cell has morphological features of a normal plasma cell. Consequently, a monoclonal immunoglobulin component (M-Ig) of a concentration usually less than 0.5 mg/ml can be detected in the serum. It persists for months, usually till the death of the animal. The isotype of M-Ig is mostly IgG (IgG2a subclass being most frequent in the C57BL mice), but M-Ig of IgM and less frequently IgA have also been observed. The concentration of the other, uninvolved Ig is usually not clearly affected. Production of a Bence-Jones protein in excess has not yet been observed in mice with BMG.
When transplanted into normal syngeneic recipient mice, the BMG clone shows 'take', expands, levels-off and persists thereafter at about the same or smaller size as in the donor mouse. In subsequent transplantations, however, the 'take' frequency of BMG decreases and propagation of the clone for more than 3 to 4 generations was never achieved. Studies on factors influencing the development of BMG demonstrated that a deficiency in the T immune system (especially in its regulatory functions) and genetic factors play an important role. Strong indication for factors bound to the C57BL genetic material has been obtained in comparative studies on the appearance of BMG in different strains, in radiation chimeras and in (C57BL x CBA)F1 mice (Radl et al.,1978; 1984; 1985). Further studies in H2 and Igh congenic C57BL and BALB strains (v.d.Akker et al., 1987; 1988) have shown that these genetic influences in the pathogenesis of BMG are complex and can not simply be ascribed to a certain H2 or Igh locus. The H2 complex did not clearly and the Igh did only to a limited extent contribute to the development of BMG. It is likely

that a defect in other subcellular C57BL related genetic factors which regulate B-cell proliferation (such as activated oncogenes) will be shown to play a more important role in this respect. Finally, intensive antigenic stimulation of mice at a young age was followed by an increased frequency of BMG; some of the M-Ig showed an antibody activity to the corresponding antigen. This indicates that memory cells may become targets of the events leading to the development of BMG.

MULTIPLE MYELOMA

The mouse MM of spontaneous origin (the 5T MM series) so far consist of 10 cases. Their major clinical and laboratory findings have been described in detail and reviewed previously (Radl et al. 1988). They are briefly summarized in table 1. Most of the 5T MM have been propagated by transplantation and form stable lines, changing very little with time. It is interesting that this limited number of MM consists of a wide spectrum of neoplasias clearly differing by their clinical course: from a very aggressive form with short survival of the mice, to a slowly growing, relatively benign MM which is comparable to the so called 'smoldering' myeloma (SMM) as described in man (Kyle, 1980). However, all of the 5T MM are transplantable with a high 'take' frequency for an unlimited number of generations.

IS THERE A RELATIONSHIP BETWEEN BMG AND MM ?

For a long time, this question has been central in a dispute among clinicians. Some authors consider BMG and MM as two different entities, stressing that BMG is essentially a benign condition. Others, using the terms BMG and MGUS (monoclonal gammopathy of undetermined significance) without a distinction, believe that BMG represents a pre-malignant condition, a pre-myeloma. This dispute is not only academic; in practice, in extremes, the latter ideas may lead to unnecessary repeated x-ray examinations of the bones or even to treatment of a possibly benign condition with cytostatics . If we assume that BMG and MM in the C57BL mice are very similar to or identical with those in man, the answer to the above question will be as follows:

1. BMG and MM are two different entities. As demonstrated in transplantation studies (Radl et al.1979, 1988), the clonal cells of both proliferative disorders show an autonomous growth, but they differ (apart from some other less pronounced features) in one most essential property, i.e. the mortality of the cell: only the MM (including SMM) cell is immortal.

2. It is unlikely that BMG represents a pre-myeloma condition. Should that be the case, MM will be expected to develop from BMG more frequently than from a normal B cell. In the aging C57BL mice, more than 80% of mice develop BMG. From the ten 5T MM, a detailed follow-up of the primary form was available in five cases. In each case, the MM developed de novo and not from a pre-existing monoclonal gammapathy with characteristics of BMG.

Table 1. **THE MOUSE 5T MULTIPLE MYELOMA SERIES**
Biological features and comparison with human disease

Features:	Human MM	5T MM primary	5T MM transpl.	Remark:
Spontaneous origin	+	+	-	
Frequency age-related	+	+	-	
Genetic predisposition	likely	likely		
Broad spectrum of clinical course	+	+	+	from'smoldering' to p.c. leukemia
Primary localization in bone marrow	+	+	+	
Bone lesions:				
osteolytic	+	+	+	
osteosclerotic	rare		rare	
Anemia	+	+	+	
Myeloma kidney	+		rare	5T2 MM
Sensitivity to chemotherapy	often low		high	only 5T2 MM tested
Progressive monoclonal proliferation	+	+	+	
Atypical ("myeloma") plasma cells	+	+	+	> in transpl. form
Aneuploidy	often	?	often	
Intraclonal heterogeneity	+	+	+	Ref. Croese ea 1987
c-myc oncogene rearrangement	- *	-	- *	Radl ea 1990 * very rare
Paraproteinemia	+	+	+	
progressively increasing	+	+	+	
concentration	>25mg/ml	>0.5mg/ml	>0.5mg/ml	
most frequent isotype	IgG	IgG		
subclass	IgG1	IgG2b		
light chain type	kappa	kappa		
Excess Bence Jones protein production	often	?	+	
Depression of other Ig	+	+	+	
Transplantation exp.:				
transplantable		+	+	as BMG
cell immortal		+	+	in contrast with BMG

3. However, both BMG and MM develop frequently in the same mouse strain, i.e. the C57BL mice, and not separately in different strains. This indicates a similar genetic susceptibility for the development of both disorders (see also infrequent reports on the occurence of BMG and MM in the same human families).

Coming back to the clinical dispute whether or not BMG is a pre-myeloma and why in man "some BMG" developed into a clear-cut malignancy after several years of a non-progressive course, I would like to offer a possible explanation for this latter problem. It may be that these infrequent (and not always well documented) observations were dealing not with BMG but with MM from the beginning, however in a relatively benign 'smoldering' form. It has repeatedly been demonstrated that plasmacytomas in mice remained sensitive to some regulatory influences of the (T) immune system (Lynch et al.1979, Abbas and Moser,1984). The 5T7 MM in the C57BL mice, while having all important MM properties similar to the other MM, remains very long in a non-progressive stage and eventually kills the host mice only when they begin to age. It has also been shown that with aging, especially the T (regulatory) cell functions decline. As this age-related immunodeficiency is gradually developing, it may disturb the delicate balance between the host defence mechanisms and the growth properties of the MM and allows further progression of the malignancy. Of course, there is an other alternative, that a new clonal variant appeared as a consequence of a new mutation having a growth or 'non-recognition' advantage over the original clonal MM cell.

Let us further assume that this hypothesis is correct and that the data obtained from the mouse experiments are valid also for the human situation; It still does not offer immediate help to the clinician in his daily practice. There are no good tests yet to unambiguously distinguish human BMG from SMM or WM within a short period of time. However, this knowledge obtained from experimental conditions should help to avoid unnecessary mistakes in terminology and possibly in making correct diagnosis or initiating treatment. The term BMG should be reserved to real benign conditions. Whenever the origin of a monoclonal gammapathy is not (yet) known, the tentative terms MGUS or idiopathic paraproteinaemia are more proper. One should realize that BMG is at least 100 times more frequent than MM and that the vast majority of MG fulfilling the clinical and laboratory criteria of BMG (including its stability for at least four years) will remain BMG. The results of the experiments in the C57BL mouse models should stimulate research efforts into discovering better tests for the differential diagnosis between BMG and MM. As the clonal cells of BMG and MM differ in such an essential property as is cell mortality, there should be a possibility to reveal that in a clinical laboratory. Tests for (dys)function of different (onco)genes or for different survival of cells under certain in vitro conditions seem to offer the most promising possibilities.

REFERENCES

Abbas AK, Moser C (1984) Idiotypic suppression of B-cell-derived tomors. Models for lymhocyte regulation. In: Greene MI, Nisonoff A, (eds) The biology of idiotypes, Plenum Press, New York, London, p 315-325

Croese JW, Vas Nunes CM, Radl J, van den Enden-Vieveen MHM, Brondijk RJ and Boersma WJA (1987) The 5T2 mouse multiple myeloma model: Characterization of 5T2 cells within the bone marrow. Br J Cancer 56: 555-560
Kyle RA, Greipp PR (1980) Smoldering multiple myeloma. New Engl J Med 302: 1347-1349
Lynch RG, Rohrer JW, Odermatt B, Gebel HD, Autry JR and Hoover RG (1979) Immunoregulation of murine myeloma cell growth and differentiation: a monoclonal model of B cell differentiation. Immunol Rev 48: 45-80
Radl J (1981) Benign monoclonal gammopathy (Idiopathic paraproteinemia). Amer J Pathol 105: 91-93
Radl J (1986) Benign Monoclonal Gammapathy (BMG). Current Topics Microbiol Immunol 132: 221-224
Radl J (1989) Benign Monoclonal Gammopathy. Model No 234, Supplemental Update, In: Capen CC, Jones TC and Migaki G (eds) Handbook: Animal Models of Human Disease, Fasc.17, Registry of Comparative Pathology, Washington,DC
Radl J, Hollander CF, van den Berg P, and de Glopper E (1978) Idiopathic paraproteinaemia I. Studies in an animal model - the ageing C57BL/KaLwRij mouse. Clin exp Immunol 33: 35-402
Radl J, de Glopper E, Schuit HRE and Zurcher C (1979) Idiopathic paraproteinemia II. Transplantation of the paraprotein producing clone from old to young C57BL/KaLwRij mice. J Immunol 122: 609-613
Radl J, Heidt PJ, Knaan-Shanzer S and van Zwieten MJ (1984) Idiopathic paraproteinaemia IV. The role of genetic factors in the development of monoclonal B cell proliferative disorders - a study in the ageing C57BL/KaLwRij and CBA/BrARij mouse radiation chimeras. Clin exp Immunol 57: 213-216
Radl J, van den Enden-Vieveen MHM, van den Akker ThW, Benner R, Haaijman JJ and Zurcher C (1985) Idiopathic paraproteinaemia V. Expression of Igh1 and Igh5 allotypes within the homogeneous immunoglobulins of ageing (C57BL/LiARij x CBA/BrARij)F1 mouse. Clin exp Immunol 62: 405-411
Radl J, Croese JW, Zurcher C, van den Enden-Vieveen MHM and de Leeuw AM (1988) Animal Model of Human Disease: Multiple Myeloma. Amer J Pathol 132: 593-597
Radl J, van den Enden-Vieveen MHM, Zurcher C, Roholl PJM and Blauw E. (1989) Morbus Waldenström-like lymphoma in the aging C57BL/KaLwRij mouse. In: Radl J and van Camp B (eds) Monoclonal Gammapathies - Clinical significance and basic mechanisms. Vol.12, Topics in Aging Research in Europe, Eurage, Rijswijk, p 233-238
Radl J, Punt YA, van den Enden-Vieveen MHM, Bentvelzen PAJ Bakkus MHC, van den Akker TW and Benner R (1990) The 5T mouse multiple myeloma model: absence of c-myc oncogene rearrangement in early transplant generations. Br J Cancer 61: 276-278
Van den Akker ThW, Tio-Gillen AP, Benner R, Zurcher C and Radl J (1987) The influence of H-2 genetic factors on the development of benign monoclonal gammopathy in ageing H-2 congenic C57BL and BALB mice. Immunology, 61: 403-408
Van den Akker ThW, de Glopper-van den Veer E, Radl J and Benner R. (1988) The influence of genetic factors associated with the immunoglobulin heavy chain locus on the development of benign monoclonal gammapathy in aging Igh congenic mice. Immunology 65: 31-35

Louvain Rats and Their Immunocytomas

H. Bazin

Experimental Immunology Unit, Faculty of Medicine, University of Louvain, Clos Chapelle aux Champs 30.56
B-1200 Brussels, Belgium

INTRODUCTION

Tumors secreting large quantities of immunoglobulins have always focused the attention of scientists as their secreted products are a convenient source of reagents and an indicator of the vitality of the tumoral cells.
Laboratory animals have supplied immunologists with an especially useful model, the BALB/c plasmacytoma model (Potter, 1972). Another interesting model is the LOUVAIN rat immunocytomas which have provided myeloma proteins of eight different (sub)isotypes and two classes of light chain in the rat and particularly the first IgD and IgE monoclonal immunoglobulins identified in an animal species. This model has also been interesting for it has provided a fusion cell line for rat hybridomas (Galfré et al.,1979;Bazin, 1990) and a model of c-myc immunoglobulin juxtaposition suggesting a role for this chromosomal translocation in the genesis of these tumors (Wiener et al.,1982;Pear et al.,1986a).

ILEOCECAL IMMUNOCYTOMAS IN RATS

In scientific literature, description of lymphoid tumors arising in the ileocecal area of rats has been reported since the 1930s. Over the years, these tumors have been described as lymphosarcomas or reticulum cell sarcomas and have been particularly well studied in a series of articles (Curtis and Dunning 1940; Dunning and Curtis 1946) in the U.S. and in France (Roussy and Guérin 1942; Guérin 1954) (Table 1). Probably the majority of these tumors were immunocytomas, although none of them were investigated for their immunoglobulin-secreting properties. Most important, the mean incidence of these ileocecal lymphoid tumors was always estimated to be lower than 3%.

In 1955 the attention of Joseph Maisin and his colleagues was drawn to tumors which appeared in the ileocecal region of the rats that they were studying. Some years later, they published that these tumors were secreting myeloma proteins. In 1969, we started an exhaustive study of these rat ileocecal tumors (abbreviated in IR tumors) and of the rats which develop them and which are now called LOUVAIN rats (abbreviated in LOU rats). They are easy to breed and are presently fully inbred. Two substrains of LOU rats were obtained. The LOU/C rat substrain was chosen for its high incidence of immunocytomas and the LOU/M rat substrain was selected for its reproduction rate and its low incidence of immunocytomas. These two substrains have always been kept mutually histocompatible, as shown

Table 1
Ileocecal tumors reported in rats (rattus norvegicus)

Strain	Number of animal examined	Number of animals with tumors	Number of animals with ileocecal lymphosarcoma or reticulum cell sarcoma	Incidence in total population	Reference
Wild rats	23,000	21	1	-	1
Fisher	31,868	110	41	-	2
August		92	5	-	2
Marshall		43	1	-	2
Zimmerman		31	10	-	3
Copenhagen		100	0	-	3
Thompson		2	1	-	3
Hybrids between August and Fisher strains		44	16	-	3
"A hooded strain"	Colony of 200-500 animals observed for 2½ years	-	99	-	4
Fisher line 344	-	-	-	1-1.5%	5
AxC line 9935	-	-	-	>1-1.5%	5
Wistar albino rats	83 (necropsied)	-	21	-	6
Osborne-Mendel albino rats	323	-	3	-	7
Noninbred albino rats	4,000	-	20	-	8
Wistar albinos	1,000	-	9	1%	9
Gray Norways	185	-	5	2.5%	9
Copenhagen line 2331	4,596	605	2	-	10
Fisher line 344	7,059	97	67	-	10
Hybrids between Copenhagen and Fisher strains	3,970	172	59	-	10
Osborne-Mendel	498	184	1	-	11
Long Evans strain	30	-	1	-	12
Noninbred albino rats	-	-	12	1%	13
Rochester strain of Wistar rats	786	189	23	±3%	14

[1]Wolley and Wherry (1911);[2]Bullock and Curtis (1930);[3]Curtis et al. (1931);[4]McEuen (1938,1939);[5]Curtis and Dunning (1940);[6]Jenney (1941);[7]Nelson and Morris (1941);[8]Roussy and Guérin (1942);[9]Farris and Yeakel (1944);[10]Dunning and Curtis (1946);[11]Saxton et al. (1948);[12]Moon et al. (1950);[13]Guérin (1954);[14]Crain (1958).

by indefinite acceptance of skin grafts from LOU/C on LOU/M and reciprocally. The lag period of development of their tumors is about 9 months. Their maximum incidence is between 12 and 14 months. The incidence in males is twice as high as in females. The tumor could appear up to the end of the life of these animals, at least in laboratory conditions (Fig. 1).

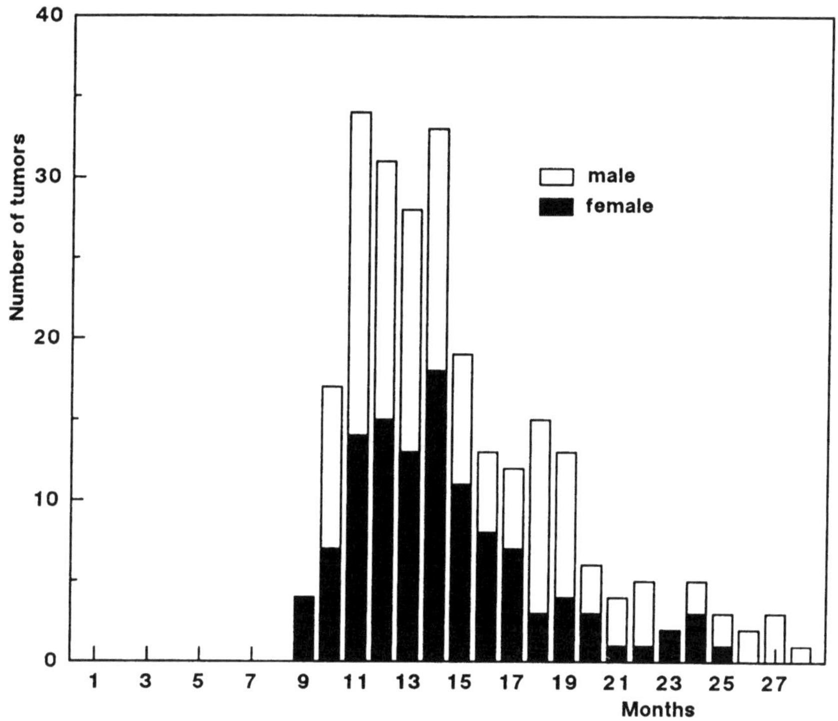

Fig.1. Age of development of spontaneous ileocecal immunocytomas in LOUVAIN rats.

MACROSCOPIC AND MICROSCOPIC ASPECTS OF THE RAT IMMUNOCYTOMAS

Generally, tumors appear in the peritoneal cavity as solid masses. They can be detected by palpation of the abdomen. Ascitic fluid is sometimes present in variable quantities which can go up to 100 ml or even more. These tumors grow very quickly in days or weeks and kill their bearers within the month of the first detection (Bazin et al., 1972).

In most cases, at autopsy the tumor is located in the ileocecal area, in the form of one, two or even three solid nodules. This location corresponds to the ileocecal lymph node, which is a group of three to five nodes; one of these nodes is generally larger than the others and is found near the cecum, the others being along the terminal ileum. They do not seem to have a special anatomy and be any different from other lymph nodes. They particularly drain the cecum, which is well developed in the rat species.

The primitive tumor seems to appear in the ileocecal lymph node and rapidly form metastasis in other places.

The histological aspect of the IR masses is characteristic of a lymphoid tumor. However, the cells cannot be described as plasma cells, but rather poorly differentiated lymphoid cells in the majority of cases. The immunoglobulin-secreting cells exhibit a granular nucleus with relatively small nuclei, a ring of deeply basophilic and pyroninophilic cytoplasm (Bazin et al. 1973; Bazin et al. 1972; Maisin et al. 1958). In immunofluorescence, with fluorescein conjugated rabbit antisera anti-rat immunoglobulin, many cells appear to have large quantities of cytoplasmic immunoglobulins. In the electron microscope, immunoglobulin-secreting tumors are polymorphic. Their nuclei are granular with very large nucleoli. Their cytoplasm is poorly basophilic with an underdeveloped endoplasmic reticulum, although ribosomes may occur in large numbers (Bazin and Beckers 1973; Burtonboy et al. 1978).

BIOSYNTHESIS OF Ig BY RAT IMMUNOCYTOMAS

Class-distribution of monoclonal immunoglobulin synthesized by IR tumors

Animals carrying an immunocytoma were killed as late as possible and both their sera and urine were analyzed for monoclonal immunoglobulins. From 1168 immunocytomas obtained to date in our rat colony of LOU/C, LOU/M, and Louvain F1 hybrids, 20 tumors were not classified, as the rats in which these tumors were discovered were in poor condition; 383 were not secreting and 765 were secreting complete immunoglobulin molecules with or without Bence-Jones proteins (Table 2). Table 3 gives the distribution of serum monoclonal immunoglobulins and Bence-Jones (BJ) proteins synthesized by 250 immunocytomas which appeared consecutively in our LOUVAIN rat colony. The class distribution of 758 secreting IR tumors is given in Table 4. This class distribution was found to be very similar for monoclonal immunoglobulins synthesized by the pure Louvain IR tumors or by IR tumors which appeared in various crosses of these rats with different inbred rat strains (Carter and Bazin 1980).

Table 2
Immunoglobulin-secreting properties of 1163 immunocytomas

	Total immunocytomas	Not determined	Nonsecreting tumor	Secreting tumor
No.	1168	20	383	765
%	100	1.7	32.4	65.4

Table 3
Distribution of the monoclonal immunoglobulins synthesized by 250 consecutive Louvain immunocytomas

	Secreting tumors	Monoclonal with or without BJ proteins	BJ proteins only
No. IR tumors	185	159	26
Absolute %	74	64	10
% secreting tumors	100	86	14

Table 4
Class distribution of the monoclonal immunoglobulins synthesized by 758 immunocytomas

	Secreting tumors	IgM	IgD	IgG1	IgG2a	IgG2b	IgG2c	IgE	IgA
No.	759	24	6	261	50	4	37	343	34
%	100	3.16	.79	34.38	6.59	.53	4.87	45.19	4.48

Clearly the mouse and rat models differ from each other, the monoclonal immunoglobulins produced by the BALB/c mice being predominantly of the IgA isotype and those by the Louvain rats of the IgE isotype.

Synthesis of monoclonal immunoglobulins by the immunocytomas

In rats bearing primitive immunocytomas the serum levels of monoclonal immunoglobulin were found to be quite variable. An example is given in Bazin and Beckers (1976) concerning the IgE isotype: IgE serum levels were found to be from 1 to 37 mg/ml, the majority of the titers being around 10 mg/ml. Beckers and Bazin (1978) gave serum level titrations for the other immunoglobulin isotypes, showing that these levels could be very high in some cases. As usual in such immunoglobulin-secreting tumors, the serum levels of the normal polyclonal immunoglobulin were all lower than in the control animal (H. Bazin, unpublished results).

The properties of the Louvain immunocytomas which secrete monoclonal immunoglobulins, when transplanted, are quite variable. Most of the IgM- or IgG-secreting tumors retain their properties for years. IgE and IgD tumors seem to be more prone to losing their secreting properties, but good producers have been obtained for all isotypes.

Antigen-binding properties

Two monoclonal immunoglobulins of the IgM (IR473) and of the IgA (IR22) isotypes, respectively, have been found to have rheumatoid factor properties for rat IgG1 molecules. No other binding capacities have been identified, particularly for the common antigens (kindly given by M. Potter, National Institute of Health,

Bethesda, Maryland) found capable of binding to BALB/c monoclonal proteins.

TRANSPLANTATION, IN VITRO CULTURE, AND STORAGE OF RAT IMMUNOCYTOMAS

In vivo transplantation

From 90 to 95% of the primitive Louvain immunocytomas can be transplanted in histocompatible animals. The tumor is removed under clean conditions and teased apart in a Petri dish. The tumor tissue is minced until it can be aspirated through a 19-gauge needle into a syringe. Between 0.1 and 0.2 ml (± 10 million cells) are injected subcutaneously into one side of the chest. After a first subcutaneous transplantation, the tumor is generally injected in the intraperitoneal cavity, using dissociated cells from the solid tumor. In nearly all cases, after a few passages, it is possible to obtain an ascitic tumor which can be transplanted by injecting 0.2-0.5 ml of ascitic fluid into the peritoneal cavity. The latent periods of transplanted Louvain immunocytomas are generally shortened after two or three passages from 14-21 days to 7-10 days. No F1 hybrid effects have been observed in inoculating small numbers of IR cells in LOU/M rats or in hybrids of first generation between this strain and rats of various other inbred strain.

In vitro cell culture

Burtonboy et al. (1973) first established continuous cell lines from immunocytomas, using the procedure established for long-term culture of hematopoietic cells of human origin (Moore et al. 1967), and found that ascitic fluid provided a more suitable starting material than cells from solid tumors. Later, Bennich et al. (1978) adapted the IR2 and IR162 IgE-secreting immunocytomas to in vitro culture and Bazin (unpublished results) adapted a dozen IR tumors to in vitro culture. Two tumors have been particularly cultivated as a fusion line for obtaining of rat-rat hybridomas: the first one, the S210 cell line, a kappa Bence-Jones producer (Bazin et al. 1972), was adapted to in vitro culture by Burtonboy et al. (1973) and given to C. Milstein and then called Y3 Ag1,2,3 (Galfré et al. 1979); the second one, IR983F, a nonsecreting cell line, was adapted to cell culture from the IR983 tumor by Bazin (1981,1982). In most of the cases, the IR tumors can easily be adapted to in vitro cell culture using conventional technology (Bazin 1982; Bazin 1986; De Clercq et al. 1986).

Storage

Louvain immunocytomas can easily be stored in liquid nitrogen as described by Bazin et al. (1972). Primitive tumors, kept for a continuous period of 14 years in liquid nitrogen, have been transplanted in histocompatible animals, and three out of four were recovered. Immunocytoma cells adapted to in vitro culture can also be frozen as described by Bazin (1987) for rat-rat hybridoma cells and kept in liquid nitrogen for years.

ETIOLOGY OF THE LOU/C RAT IMMUNOCYTOMAS

Genetic control

It has been shown that, in the same conditions of breeding, clear difference in immunocytoma incidence in various inbred strains of rat: LOU/C rats may have a high incidence, LOU/M, AUG and AxC, a low or a very low incidence and the OKA rats, a nil incidence (Beckers and Bazin, 1978). An intermediate incidence has been found in hybrids obtained by crossing LOU/C and AUG, AxC or LOU/M rats, whatever the strains of the male or female taken to make the hybrids. By contrast (LOU/C x OKA)F1 had a very low incidence of 1.08% (Bazin et al., 1987). This resistance was not linked to special properties of the immunoglobulin genes of the OKA strains as congenic rats having respectively the kappa or the heavy chains of immunoglobulins of the OKA strain in the LOU/C genetic background, have a tumor incidence identical to the LOU/C strain. The LOU/C.Rt-1^{k} (OKA), congenic to the LOU/C rats, having the OKA haplotype of the major histocompatibility complex in the LOU/C genetic background showed no immunocytoma incidence, indicating that the OKA MHC or genes linked to it determines resistance to immunocytoma appearance.

Chromosomal translocation in the immunocytomas

Chromosomal translocation is consistently associated with a variety of hematopoietic malignancies. Particularly, studies on Burkitt's lymphoma and pristane induced mouse plasmacytomas have shown that c-myc is involved in a reciprocal exchange with one of the three immunoglobulin loci in 100% of the cases.

Wiener et al. (1982) and Pear et al. (1988a) have detected a consistent translocation in early passage LOU/C immunocytomas arising from a reciprocal exchange between the distal part of the q-arm of chromosome 7 and the telomeric region of chromosome 6 with breakpoints at 7 q 3.3 and 6 q 3.2, respectively. A detailled analysis of these translocations have been made by G. Klein and his colleagues, F. Wiener, W.S. Pear, J. Sumegi (Sumegi et al., 1983; Pear et al., 1986a,b;1988b) concluding that the same genetic loci were juxtaposed by chromosomal translocation in the LOU immunocytomas as in the Burkitt's lymphomas and mouse plasmacytomas.

Modification of the immunocytoma incidence

Attempts were made to modify the incidence or the latent period of the immunocytoma in LOU/C rats.

By removing the ileocecal lymph nodes of 5 to 21 day-old rats, Moriamé et al. (1977) were able to considerably decrease the immunocytoma incidence of LOU/C rats as compared to their controls. On the contrary, no increase has never been obtained by local or total irradiation, injection of irritating substances in the peritoneal cavity.

Evolution of the immunocytoma incidence in function of time

The incidence of the rat lymphoid ileocecal tumor is quite intriguing. In the literature, observation of the appearance and disappearance of such tumors has been described.

"Since the beginning of 1936, a lymphosarcoma originating in the ileocecal mesenteric lymph nodes had made its appearance in the colony" wrote McEuen, 1938. However, at least a case is quoted in which the propensity to develop such tumors disappeared in a colony: Gilbert et al. (1958) explained "in respect to the lymphosarcoma, the Utrecht strain rats undoubtedly were akin to the rats of Curtis et al. (1931). But this kinship was altered in the first generation of Utrecht rats when the frequency of lymphosarcoma was sharply reduced to 2.2% and to 0% in the second and subsequent generations".

About 1955, it was noted (Maisin et al., 1955a and b) that some of non inbred ancestors of the LOUVAIN rats developed tumors arising from the ileocecal lymph node area. At that time, the incidence of these tumors was around 1-3%.

In the early seventies, when we began to breed these rats, their immunocytoma incidence had seemed to rise markedly, so as to exceed the 10% level and even later 30% in male and 15% in female, possibly on account of selection of breeders from litters with high tumor frequency.

As an example, Figure 2 gives the pedigree of a family of LOU/C rats during 27 generations. It shows an appearance of tumor at generation 5 and a disappearance at generation 24. However, it can be noted that many generations between these two were without tumor development. Moreover, the tumor incidence is normal in the male (around 30%) but particularly low in the female.

Historically, we began with 28 different and distinct lines of rats coming from the various colonies kept in the University of LOUVAIN. We observed their tumor incidence in the ileocecal area. The line presenting the highest incidence in ileocecal tumor was chosen as histocompatibility reference for the model and called LOU/C. The line presenting the lowest incidence of ileocecal tumor and a histocompatibility identical to the LOU/C rats as judged by reciprocal skin grafts was called LOU/M.
In 1976, six distinct lines of LOU/C rats were selected and developed; we were always trying to select the breeder rats from the line or the family having a high incidence of ileocecal tumor.

However, some years later, as seen in Figure 3, we were obliged to decrease the size of our rat colony due to a decrease in our financial support. Moreover, in 1982, we discovered a viral infection in our colony and were obliged to caesarian derive our rat strains and to disinfect our animal house. At that time, our colony of LOU/C rats was reduced to a single couple. Since that time, we have kept a low number of animals under observation, and we still have a low incidence in immunocytomas, but it is much lower than the previous one.

Which are the etiological factors of the immunocytoma incidence in the rat species and especially in the LOUVAIN strain?

A special genetic background is certainly important. Some strains seem susceptible, some others, resistant. Since 1975-76 at least, the LOU/C strain has been totally inbred. Its high immunocytoma incidence could be linked to a peculiar characteristic specific to this strain or to the selection that we have realized in our colony during a period of time. On the contrary, some strains, like the OKA are resistant, the resistance gene being linked to the major histocompatibility complex.

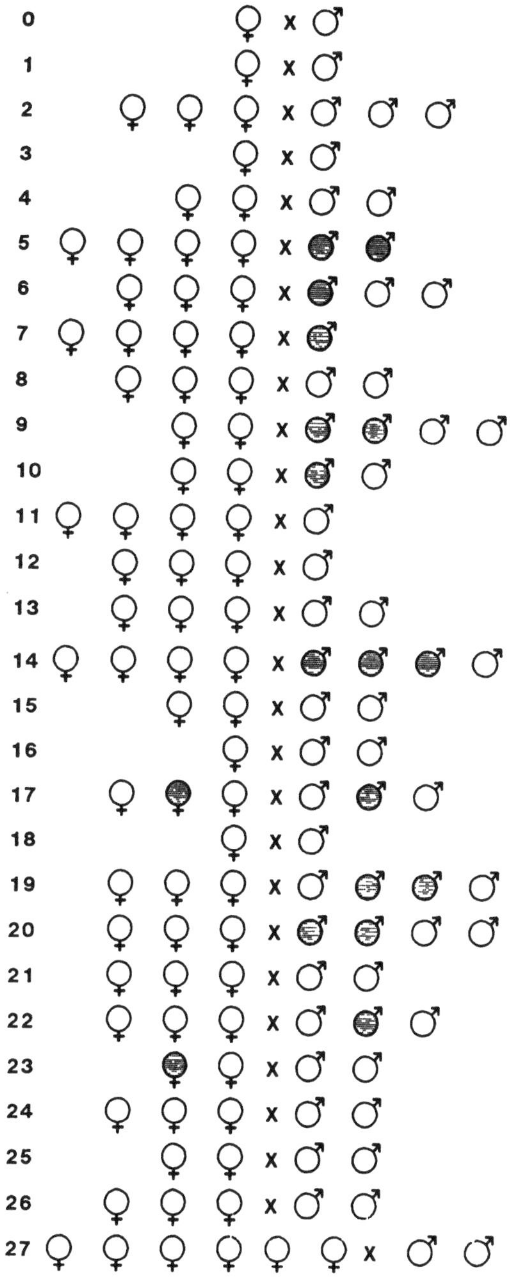

Figure 2

The pedigree of a LOU/C family during 27 generations, ending in 1983. The open circles correspond to rat without immunocytoma, the close circle, to rats having developed an immunocytoma. The numbers, at left, are the generations.

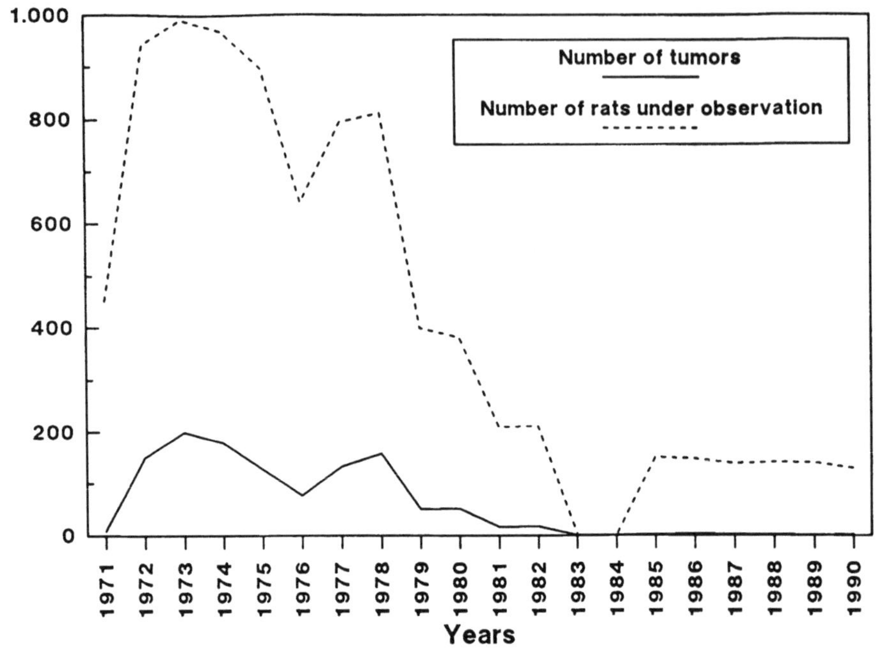

Figure 3

Number of immunocytomas observed in our LOU/C colony as well as the number of rats under observation, in function of years.

But a special genetic background is certainly not enough to get a special incidence, as it disappeared at the time of caesarian derivation, and the cleaning of our animal house. What could be this special factor? By keeping together in the same cage, LOU/C and susceptible rats, like LOU/M or August or AxC rats, horizontal transmission of the immunocytoma incidence has never appeared, but by mating these animals, an incidence approximately equal to half those of the two strains, has been obtained.

The percentage of LOUVAIN immunocytomas being very high in IgE secreting tumors, we have tried to infect some of our LOU/C rats, with larvae of Siphasia, a common helminth of the rat species which lives in the caecum and which, as all helminthes, particularly stimulates the IgE production of the host. We have obtained no increase in our basic tumor incidence. In fact, the only change that we have obtained in this tumor incidence, has been a decrease after surgical removal of the ileocecal lymph nodes in newborn LOU/C rats. A possible explanation of this result could be the dilution of a factor coming from the caecum, by the lymph route and reaching at first, the ileocecal nodes. The disappearance of these nodes can possibly lead to a dilution of this hypothetic factor under a limit concentration when reaching the next lymph nodes.

However, quite clearly up to now, we have not found the etiological factors of the LOUVAIN rat immunocytomas and are still looking for them.

CONCLUSION

We have obtained, in about ten years, eleven hundred tumors called immunocytomas, they had a high aggressivity for their hosts, very often giving large amounts of monoclonal immunoglobulins, able to be tranplanted from animal to animal in the same strain and to be adapted to in vitro culture. These tumors have all an already identified chromosomal translocation activating the c-myc oncogene. However, this oncogene activation is not the only etiological cause for this tumor incidence. From one to three per cent of rats, in some defined strains, can get such tumors, probably in special environment giving enough antigenic stimulations.

It is possible that, by selecting animals in parallel lines having the highest incidence of such immunocytomas, we have been able to increase the percentage of tumors up to 30% in male and 15% in female. However, limiting our colony, we lost this incidence, which is back to the former. Unfortunately, we still do not know which is the (co)factor responsible for this tumor appearance.

REFERENCES

Bazin H (1981) Les anticorps monoclonaux. Louvain Medical 100:3-8.

Bazin H (1982 Production of rat monoclonal antibodies with the LOU rat non secreting IR983F myeloma cell line. In: Peeters E (ed) Protides of the biological fluids, Pergamon Press, Oxford and N.Y., p 615-618.

Bazin H (1987) Rat-rat hybridoma formation and rat monoclonal antibodies. In: Bartal AH, Hirshaut Y, Methods of Hybridoma Formation, Humana Press, Clifton, New Jersey, p 337-378.

Bazin H, ed. (1990) Rat Hybridomas and Rat Monoclonal Antibodies. CRC Press Inc., Boca Raton, USA, 515 pages.

Bazin H, Beckers A (1976) Nobel Symposium 33, Molecular and biological aspects of the acute allergic reaction. In: Johanson SGO, Stranberg K, Uvnas B (eds), Plenum Company, New York, p 125-151.

Bazin H, Beckers A, Deckers C, Moriamé M (1973) Tranplantable immunoglobulin-secreting tumours in rats. V. Monoclonal immunoglobulins secreted by 250 ileocecal immunocytomas in the LOU/Wsl rats. J Natl Cancer Inst 51:1359-1361.

Bazin H, Deckers C, Beckers A, Heremans JF (1972) Transplantable immunoglobulin-secreting tumours in rats.I.General features in LOU/Wsl strain rat immunocytomas and their monoclonal proteins. Int J Cancer, 10:568-580.

Bazin H, Pear WS, Sumegi J (1987) LOUVAIN rat immunocytomas. Adv Cancer Res 50: 279-310.

Beckers A, Bazin H (1978) Incidence of spontaneous immunocytomas in hybrids of LOU/C rats and rat strains with spontaneous tumor incidence. J Natl Cancer Inst 60: 1505-1508.

Bennich H, Karlsson T, Bazin H, Zeuthen J (1978) In vitro culture of IgE secreting cells from two rat myelomas. Prot Biol Fluids 25:559-562.

Bullock FD, Curtis MR (1930) Spontaneous tumors of the rat. J Cancer Res 14: 1-115.

Burtonboy G, Bazin H, Deckers C, Lamy M, Heremans JF (1973) Transplantable immunoglobulin-secreting tumours in rats. III. Establishment of immunoglobulin-secreting cell lines from LOU/Wsl strain rats. Eur J Cancer 9:259-262.

Burtonboy G, Beckers A, Rodhain J, Bazin H, Lamy M (1978) Rat ileocecal immunocytomas. An ultrastructural study with special attention to the presence of viral particles. J Natl Cancer Inst 61: 477-484.

Carter P, Bazin H (1980) Immunology. In: The Laboratory Rat, vol 2, Academic Press, New York, p 182-212.

Crain RC (1958) Spontaneous tumors in the Rochester strain of the Wistar rat. Am J Pathol 34:311-323.

Curtis MR, Bullock FD, Dunning WF (1931) A statistical study of the occurrence of spontaneous tumors in a large colony of rats. Am J Cancer 40:299-309.

Curtis MR, Dunning WF (1940) Transplantable lymphosarcoma of the mesenteric lymph nodes of rats. Am J Cancer 40:299-309.

De Clercq L, Cormont F, Bazin H (1986). The use of rat monoclonal antibodies to characterize, quantify and purify polyclonal or monoclonal mouse IgM. Methods Enzymol 121: 622-631.

Dunning WF, Curtis MR (1946) The respective roles of longevity and genetic specificity in the occurrence of spontaenous tumors in the hybrids between two inbred lines of rats. Cancer 6:61-81.

Farris EJ, Yeakel EH (1944) Sponteanous and transplanted reticulum cell sarcomas in Wistar rats. Am J Pathol 20:733-781.

Galfré G, Milstein C, Wright B (1979) Rat x rat hybrid myelomas and a monoclonal anti-Fd portion of mouse IgG. Nature (London) 277: 131-133.

Gilbert C, Gillman J, Loustalot P, Lutz W (1958) The modifying influence of diet and the physical environment on spontaneous tumour frequency in rats. Brit J Cancer 12: 565-593.

Guérin M (1954) Tumeurs spontanées des animaux de laboratoire. Legrand A et Cie, Paris.

Jenney FS (1941) Reticulum cell sarcoma in the rat transferred through twelve successive passages in animals of related stock. Cancer Res 1:407-409.

Maisin J, Maisin H, Dunjic A, Maldague P (1955a) La radiobiologie comme méthode de travail en physiopathologie et en cancérologie expérimentale. Bull Acad Suisse Sci Med 11: 247-273.

Maisin J, Maldague P, Maisin H, Dunjic A (1955b) Au sujet de l'influence cancérigène de l'irradiation in toto à dose unique. CR Soc Biol (Paris) 149: 1052-1055.

Maisin J, Maldague P, Dunic A, Hong-Que P, Maisin H (1958) Le leucosarcome chez le rat. L'incidence de ce néoplasme après irradiation totale, subtotale et locale. Sang 24: 751-763.

McEuen CS (1938) Occurrence of cancer in rats treated with oestrone. Am J Cancer 34:184-195.

McEuen CS (1939) The occurrence of lymphosarcoma in rats. Am J Cancer 36:383-985.

Moon HD, Simpson ME, Li CH, Evans HM (1950) Neoplasms in rats treated with pituitary growth hormone. I. Pulmonary and lymphatic tissues. Cancer Res 10:297-308.

Moore GE, Garner RE, Franklin HA (1967) Culture of normal human leucocytes. J Am Med Assoc 199:87.

Moriamé M, Beckers A, Bazin H (1977) Decrease of the incidence of malignant ileocecal immunocytoma in LOU/C rats after surgical removal of the ileocecal lymph nodes. Cancer Lett 3: 139-143.

Nelson AA, Morris HJ (1941) Reticulum cell lymphosarcoma in rats. Arch Pathol 3: 578-584.

Pear WS, Ingvarsson S, Steffen D, Munke M, Francke U, Bazin H, Klein G, Sumegi J (1986a) Multiple chromosomal rearrangements in a spontaneously arising t(6:7) rat immunocytoma juxtapose c-myc and immunoglobulin heavy chain sequences. Proc Natl Acad Sci (US) 83:7376-7380.

Pear WS, Nelson SF, Axelsson H, Wahlström G, Bazin H, Klein G, Sumegi J (1988a) Aberrant class switching juxtaposes c-myc with a middle repetitive element (LINE) and a IgH intron in two spontaneously arising rat immunocytomas. Oncogene 2:499-507.
Pear WS, Wahlström G, Nelson SF, Axelsson H, Szles A, Wiener F, Bazin H, Klein G, Sumegi J (1988b) The 6:7 chromosomal translocation in spontaneously arising rat immunocytomas: evidence for c-myc breakpoint clustering and correlation between isotypic expression and c-myc target. Mol Cell Biol 8:441-451.
Pear WS, Wahlström G, Szpirer J, Levan G, Klein G, Sumegi J (1986b) Localization of the rat immunoglobulin heavy chain locus to chromosome 6. Immunogenetics 23: 393-395.
Potter M (1972) Immunoglobulin producing tumors and myeloma proteins of mice. Physiol Rev, 52:631-719.
Roussy G, Guérin P (1942) Les lymphosarcomes du rat. Bull Assoc Fr Etude Cancer 30:17-28.
Saxton JA, Sperling GA, Barnes LL, McCay CM (1948) The influence of nutrition upon the incidence of spontaneous tumors of the albino rat. Acta Unio Int Cancerum 6:423-431.
Sumegi J, Spira J, Bazin H, Szpirer J, Levan G, Klein G (1983) Rat c-myc oncogene is located on chromosome 7 and rearranges in immunocytomas with a t(6:) translocation. Nature 306:494-498.
Wiener F, Babonits M, Spira J, Klein G, Bazin H (1982) Non-random chromosomal changes involving chromosomes 6 and 7 in spontaneous rat immunocytomas. Int J Cancer 29:431-437.
Woolley PG, Wherry WB (1911) Notes on twenty-two spontaneous tumors in wild rats (M. Norvegicus). J Med Res 25: 205-215.

ACKNOWLEDGMENTS

I am especially indebted to the "Fonds Cancérologique de la Caisse Générale d'Epargne et de Retraite" (Belgium) for their financial support and also to the European Communities of which I am a scientific staff member (Publication No. 2547).

Induced Plasmacytoma Formation in Mice

M. Potter, E.B. Mushinski, J. Wax, and L.G. Byrd

Laboratory of Genetics, National Cancer Institute, National Institutes of Health, Bethesda, MD 20892 USA

Although plasmacytomas can develop spontaneously in mice, the more common origin requires inducing agents. In the system which we will describe, plasmacytomagenesis is initiated by the intraperitoneal injection of paraffin oils such as the alkane pristane (2,6,10,14-tetramethylpentadecane) (Anderson and Potter 1969). These tumors can also be induced by the intraperitoneal implantation of solid plastic materials as was originally discovered by Merwin and Algire (see Merwin et al. 1963). An important characteristic of plasmacytoma induction in mice is that it only works in certain inbred strains such as BALB/cAn in which the expected average incidence is ~ 60%, or NZB where between 30 and 40% of the mice develop these tumors; most other inbred strains do not develop these tumors (Morse et al. 1980). Plasmacytomas have been studied cytogentically by Francis Wiener and Shinsuke Ohno, and over 95% of them have reciprocal chromosomal translocations involving immunoglobulin genes (chromosomes 12 and 6 and 16) and c-myc (chromosome 15) or loci near c-myc such as Pvt-1 (Ohno et al. 1979,1984). These translocations cause deregulation of c-myc transcription (Mushinski 1988). Deregulation of c-myc cooperates with other oncogenic mutations to transform certain B-lymphocytes but does not appear to be sufficient by itself to cause transformation (see Potter 1990). C-myc deregulation is consistently found in spontaneous rat immunocytomas (plasma cell tumors) and in Burkitt's lymphoma in man (see Potter 1990).

PRE-NEOPLASTIC PROLIFERATIONS OF PLASMA CELLS IN OIL GRANULOMA

The common factor among the non-viral plasmacytoma inducing agents appears to reside in their ability to induce chronic peritoneal inflammation. Moreover plasmacytomas arise directly in the inflammatory tissues induced by these agents. The relationship of plasmacytomagenesis to the inflammatory changes has not been extensively investigated for the solid plastic agents as these produce very complex changes in the peritoneum, but has been studied in some detail with paraffin oils (Potter and MacCardle 1964; Anderson et al. 1985).

Paraffin oils induce the formation of an oil granuloma (OG) on peritoneal surfaces (Potter and MacCardle 1964; Anderson et al. 1985; Leak et al. 1985) including the mesenteries of the intestine, the omentum, the connective tissue around the pancreas, pelvic tissues and fat pads, the diaphram and abdominal wall and even extends retroperitoneally to the tissues around the kidney. Large amounts of oil surrounded by macrophages and neutrophils are deposited onto peritoneal surfaces and this process is associated with an increase in the supportive tissues of the peritoneum, i.e., blood vessels and connective tissue stromal cells.

The pristane induced plasmacytomas have a long latent period of at least 120 days (a few have recently been found earlier; B. Mock, NCI personal communication) and with a mean incidence between 210 and 220 days (Potter and Wax 1983). The OG begins forming almost immediately after injection of the oil. As the plasmacytomas develop in this tissue, it is possible to examine histologically the early stages of this developmental process. In most mice, it is not difficult to find scattered solitary plasma cells throughout the OG; however, clusters of plasma cells begin to appear in some mice as soon as 25 days after the injection of oil (Potter et al. 1985). Some of these become quite large, containing 50 to several hundred plasma cells in a field that is 0.025mme2 to 0.05mme2. The plasma cells in these foci are usually hyperchromatic, frequently have an atypical distribution of chromatin in the nucleus, and exhibit mitotic figures. Foci vary in size and can become quite extensive; a few of them can even be called 'megafoci' because they contain over 500 cells. It is very difficult to accurately quantify the number of foci per mouse without doing serial sections on a large amount of tissue; however one can obtain an estimate of the number of foci by scanning the cross-sections of fragments of the entire mesentery, omentum, and available fatty tissue in the peritoneum.

In some foci the plasma cells are compactly clustered together; in others the cells appear to diffusely invade a sector of the mesenteric OG and can be found along blood vessels or in the planes between mesenteric adipose tissue and overlying OG. Also, foci can be located on the peritoneal surfaces of the mesenteric OG. In a single mouse there are frequently multiple foci that vary in their location relative to mesenteric connective tissues, the OG-tissue itself and developed plasmacytoma, the OG which initially contained a predominance of macrophages, is largely replaced by plasma cells and free tumor cells can be usually aspirated from the peritoneal space.

A major question we have considered is whether the multiple foci found in early cases, i.e., where there were 5 to 10 foci in one mouse represent multiple autochthonous developing tumors or whether the cells in a single focus spread to different sectors of the peritoneal oil granuloma. By using <u>in situ</u> (immunoperoxidase) labelling of cells, we have found that in the majority of mice with multiple foci, all of the foci are of the same heavy chain isotype. The majority of foci contain only IgA secreting cells. In some mice more than one isotype can be identified. Convincing evidence for clonality requires the use of serological idiotypic markers but these are difficult to develop for a specific tumor because the early stages of plasmacytoma formation cannot as yet be detected and isolated. One can take advantage however of rarely expressed markers for both immunoglobulin C- or V-regions; one of these is the lambda light chain. Lambda is expressed in approximately 3% of

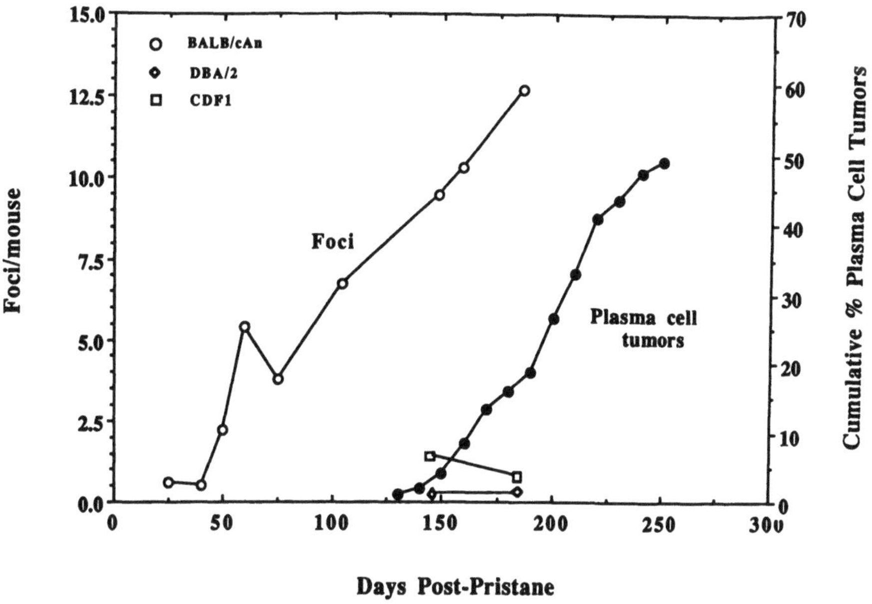

Figure 1. The estimated number of foci as a function of time.

The foci in 292 BALB/cAnPt mice from 13 experimental groups taken between days 25 and 186 and from DBA/2N and CDF1 mice at 150 and 180 days are shown. The connective tissues of the peritoneum including the mesenteries were cut in approximately 1 cme3 or smaller fragments. To enumerate the foci the sections were usually stained with methyl-green-pyronin. Mice with 25 or more foci were given a value of 25.

serum immunoglobulins (see Weiss et al. 1984) and is equally rare in myeloma proteins. We have typed the foci in 36 mice and found 3 cases in which all or a majority of foci stained with a rarely expressed light or heavy chain class. There were two lambda positive cases and one G2b. In these cases there was considerable histological variation as described above. Further, the foci appeared to be separated from each other in different regions of the mesenteries, thus suggesting that the clone had spread to different locations; rigorous proof of this point is currently being developed in our laboratory.

Most DBA/2N and (BALB/cAn x DBA/2)F1 hybrid mice that were examined between 150 and 180 days after injection of pristane did not have foci. This result indicates that predisposition to develop foci is genetically determined.

In summary, multiple foci in a single mouse appear in most cases to represent expansions of a clone of abnormally proliferating cells. Multiple foci can appear very soon after the injection of pristane, i.e., within 25 to 50 days and long before the first plasma cell tumors can be diagnosed. One of the features of plasma cell tumor development may be the time required for these initial cells to acquire the ability to spread throughout the OG and grow more autonomously.

Two points about the histogenesis of plasmacytomas in mice that may be relevant to an understanding of plasma cell tumor formation in other species are: 1) certain kinds of plasma cells, i.e., those in foci are apparently able to proliferate in the OG while many solitary plasma cells in the contiguous OG of the same mouse do not appear to be proliferating; 2) plasma cell tumors appear to evolve from these proliferating populations; and 3) the proliferating cells are very probably expansions of a single clone rather than representing a polyclonal expansion of different plasma cells. Polyclonal plasma cell proliferations may occur in such disorders as Castleman's disease or in the experimental forms of this disease that are induced by excessive IL-6 production (Suematsu et al. 1989; Brandt et al. 1990).

Are the focal plasma cell proliferations in the OG of pristane-injected mice counterparts of monoclonal gammopathies of undetermined significance (MGUS) in man? The plasma cells differ from the benign monoclonal gammopathies described by Radl and his co-workers (see Radl this volumne) by their association with an inflammatory tissue and by their appearence relatively early in life. One assumes the benign monoclonal gammopathies (BMGs) described by Radl are located in the bone marrow either as focal proliferations or as disseminated clones. A few old C57BL/KaLwRij mice do develop plasma cell tumors (Radl et al. 1988) that more closely resemble multiple myeloma in man than do the induced peritoneal plasma cell tumors in BALB/cAn mice (see Radl, this book). In five cases the 5T myeloma tumors did not develop from a pre-existing BMG. The peritoneal plasmacytomas appear, however, to evolve from abnormally proliferating precursors.

For epidemiologists, what is the fundamental lesion in multiple myeloma? Is it a predisposition to form a abnormal clone of precursor cells such as can be found in a MGUS or a focus of proliferating plasma cells in the pristane-induced OG of the BALB/cAn mouse, or is it the predisposition for a precursor lesion to progress to a malignant tumor? The predisposition to develop abnormally proliferating clones of plasma cells appears to be genetically determined. It is not clear how genes could influence this process and there may be more than one mechanism for generating such abnormal clones in mice. For example, the inbred strain which is most susceptible to peritoneal plasmacytoma development (BALB/cAn) is relatively resistant to developing BMGs (J. Radl, personal communication). This presents an intriguing problem for future research. It is also possible that the genotype of the host determines the progression of abnormal clones to an autonomous state.

THE ROLE OF ENVIRONMENTAL FACTORS IN PLASMACYTOMAGENESIS

In the BALB/cAn mouse environmental factors can influence plasmacytomagenesis. A number of years ago it was shown that less than 5% of germfree BALB/cAn mice developed plasmacytomas (McIntire and Princler 1969). This low incidence of tumors was assumed to be due to the absence of gut flora and antigenic stimulation. In a more recent study originally intended to study the role of T-cells in plasmacytomagenesis, we attempted to induce plasmacytomas in athymic BALB/cAn-nu/nu mice and found that these mice did not develop plasmacytomas either (Byrd et al. 1988). The BALB/c nude mouse congenic is maintained by breeding nu/+ x nu/nu (Fig. 2). Interestingly, the BALB/c nu/+ mice were also resistant. However, this strain was maintained in specific pathogen-free (SPF) conditions; that is, the mice were fed sterilized food and drinking water and kept in a laminar flow cabinet in cages with sterilized bedding. This result suggested that the SPF conditions like the gnotobiotic conditions might influence plasmacytomagenesis. SPF mice carry a defined bacterial flora in their gastrointestinal tracts. Accordingly, BALB/cAn-nu/+ mice were transferred to a conventional environment and after one to two generations were injected with pristane; these mice, in contrast to the SPF counterpart mice, developed plasmacytomas in the expected numbers. BALB/cAn nu/+ taken directly from the SPF cabinet and exposed to conventional conditions developed a considerably lower incidence of plasmacytomas. These results suggest that immune systems of SPF mice have not been fully activated by experiences with potential pathogens.

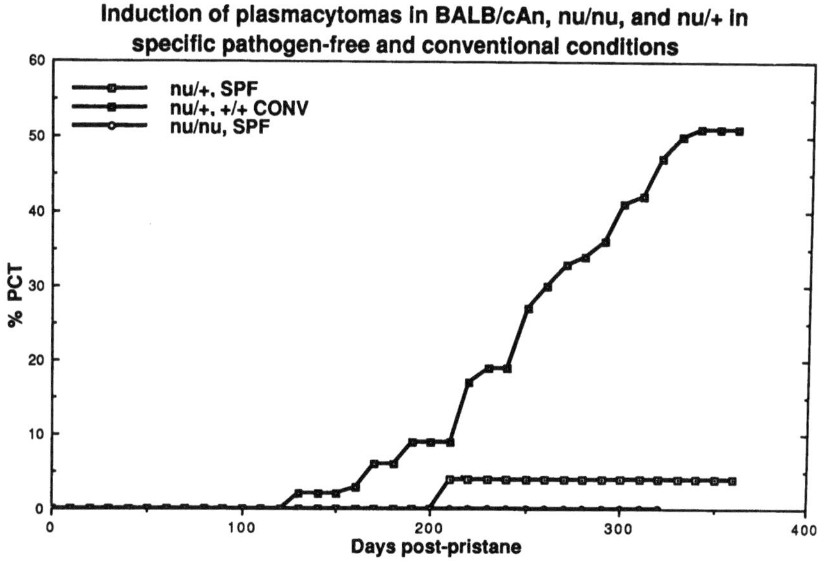

Figure 2.

The results also suggest that a relatively immunologically naive host is resistant to pristane-induced plasmacytomagenesis. Epidemiologists have questioned the possible role of specific or even multiple infections in the pathogenesis of multiple myeloma and thus far no such relationship has been found. An infection would be expected to induce a polyclonal response and possibly polyclonal antigen-driven plasma cell hyperplasias. Hyperplastic plasma cells, even including those in genetically susceptible hosts, may not be at increased risk for neoplastic development.

EFFECT OF INDOMETHACIN

The inclusion of the non-steroidal anti-inflammatory agent, indomethacin in the drinking water of pristane injected BALB/cAN mice during the latent period of plasmacytomagenesis (days 1-120) drastically reduces the formation of these tumors (Potter et al. 1985) (Fig 3). Mice given pristane in this way develop substantial tissue levels of indomethacin in the oil granuloma tissues (E. Shacter, NCI manuscript in preparation). Indomethacin treatment can be delayed until 60 days after the first injection of pristane suggesting that it can be effective in the later stages of plasma cell tumor formation, i.e., the progression from the focal plasma cell proliferation stage to overgrowth and transplantability. However, many focal plasma cell proliferations appear to develop 60 or more days after the injection of pristane and thus indomethacin could influence the development of these foci rather than their progression.

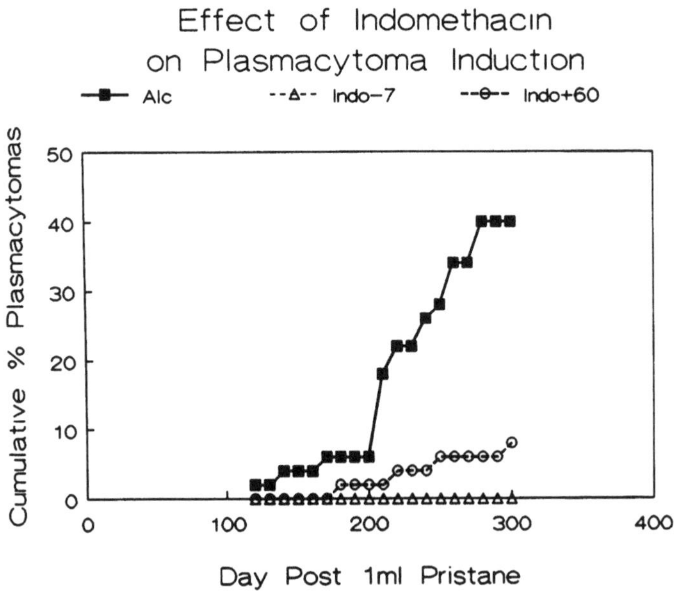

Figure 3.

Indomethacin is a powerful inhibitor of cyclo-oxygenase and blocks the formation of prostaglandins (PGs). One possibility (not substantiated as yet) is that prostaglandins are generated in higher than physiological (~10-8 M) amounts in the OG tissue (e.g., by macrophages and/or stromal cells) and that high PGE2 levels are a contributing factor to plasma cell tumor development. At this point, it must be assumed that indomethacin could act either directly by blocking endogenous PG formation in B cells or indirectly by blocking PG formation in an accessory cell.

The principle question that arises is how to explain the biological effects of PGs in plasmacytomagenesis. PGs are known to produce a number of effects on T- and B-lymphocyte proliferation and function. In general, PGs are growth inhibitory for lymphocytes. PGE2 suppresses T-lymphocyte proliferation (Goodwin et al. 1977) and the expression of IL-2 receptors in T-lymphocytes (Rincon et al. 1988). In B lymphoblasts stimulated by lipopolysaccharide (LPS), PGE2 mildly stimulates the incorporation of thymidine into DNA (Rojo et al. 1982). PGs however inhibit the maturation of certain mitogen stimulated human B lymphocytes to Ig secreting cells but apparantly do not inhibit Ig secretion itself (Jelinek et al. 1985). PGEs also inhibit the growth of certain B-cell lymphomas (Phipps et al. 1989). In the presence of certain tolerogenic agents such as heat aggregated Ig, or hapten substitutes Ig, PGE2 promotes the development of a tolerant state in B-cells (Scheuer et al. 1987; Schad and Phipps 1989; Goldings 1986); furthermore, indomethacin treatment abrogates tolerization. It would therefore appear that the principle aotion of high PG levels on B-cells may be a regulatory effect on maturation to an Ig-secreting stage. The effect on T-cells may also be regulatory and may determine the relative proportions of T-helper cells and possibly T-cytotoxic cells. The T-cell microenvironment is known to play an important role in the outcome of chronic infections such as cutaneous leishmaniasis in mice (Liew 1990). In BALB/cAn mice, which develop progressive leishmanial lesions, there is an imbalance in the relative numbers of T-helper cells (TH1 and TH2) cells. This has been attributed to the production of PGs by inflammatory macrophages (Liew 1989; Cillari et al. 1986) and also has suggested a genetically determined response in that many other strains of mice are able to resolve their lesions (Liew 1990). If similar effects that are mediated by PGs occur in the T-cells of the OG, they could potentially affect immunological surveillance and permit clonal plasma cell proliferations. In this context it can be mentioned that induced plasmacytomas are known to carry tumor associated transplantation antigens (see Potter and Walters 1973). The role of PGs in plasmacytoma development remains unknown.

THE ROLE OF GENES IN PLASMACYTOMAGENESIS

One of the intriguing biological features of the plasmacytoma induction system is that most inbred strains of mice are resistant to plasmacytomagenesis from the intraperitoneal injection of pristane. This suggests that the genotype of the host plays an important role in plasmacytoma development. In general genes could affect the character of the inflammatory tissue and hence the response of the animal to the inducing agent. Alternatively, they might act directly in B-cells. To explore the genetic basis for susceptibility (S) and resistance (R) we have studied the susceptibility of various hybrids of BALB/cAnPt (an S strain) and DBA/2NPt (an R strain) to plasmacytoma induction (see Potter 1984). The F1 hybrids (BALB/cAn x DBA/2)F1 hybrids are solidly resistant indicating that R genes are dominant. The incidence in first generation backcross to BALB/c was 11% (see Potter 1984) suggesting at least 3 loci are involved in determining the resistance of the DBA/2 mouse. These findings indicated that it would be difficult to find the genes determining susceptibility through linkage by classical Mendelian crosses. Alternatively we have attempted to find R genes by their linkage to known allelomorphic markers.

We have constructed a number of other C.D2 congenic lines and some of these are susceptible (like the BALB/cAnPt parent) but others show partial resistance. In congenic mice the resistance phenotype has thus far only been demonstrated in mice that are homozygous for putative PCT-R genes. We have focused on gene(s) located in a 30 cM distal segment of chromosome 4 (between MMTV-13 and Fv-1) in the DBA/2 mouse (Potter et al. 1984). One or more genes in this large segment determine partial resistance to plasmacytoma induction (Potter et al. 1984). This has enabled us to construct a congenic line of mice BALB/cAn.DBA/2-Fv-1 in which the Fv-1n/n marker has been introgressively backcrossed for 19 generations. The incidence of plasmacytomas in these mice is summmarized in Fig 4. A very basic question concerns the behavior of an allelomorphic R gene.

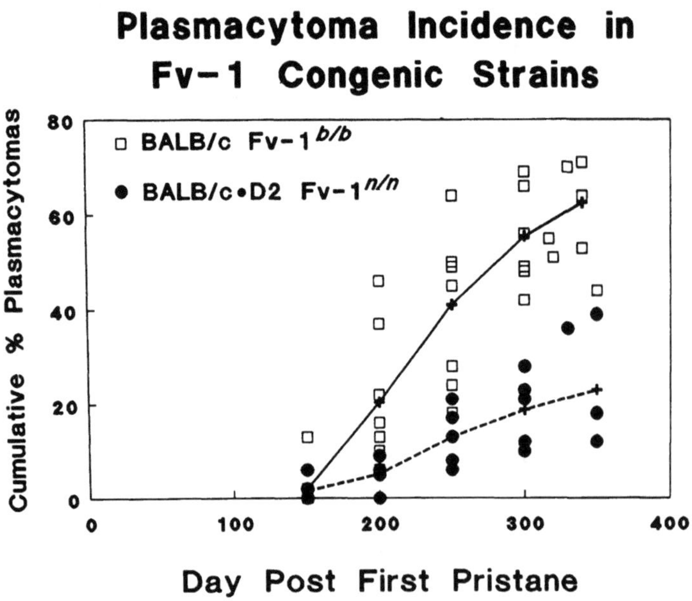

Figure 4.

Does it have strong discontinuous effects or is it more like a quantitative gene that has a realtively weak effect? As may be seen (Fig. 4), the PCT-R1 gene linked to Fv-1 determined partial resistance and hence has a quantitative rather than an all or none effect on plasmacytomagenesis. A second partial resistance gene (PCT-R2) is linked to the MHC class-I-like Qa-2 gene on chr-17. Further, when PCT-R1 genes on chr-4 and PCT-R2 on chr-17 are combined in a single congenic strain, the mice show even greater resistance (unpublished data).

Our data suggest there may be multiple genes in Mus musculus that influence susceptibility and resistance to disease. The inbreeding of mice and the establishment of inbred strains has by chance assembled in the BALB/cAn genome a number of susceptibility alleles. An assemblage of susceptibility genes may also have occurred in different races of homo sapiens for reasons not yet understood and these could play role in determining the susceptibility to develop MGUS and multiple myeloma in man. Because susceptibility genes are multiple and have quantitative effects they may be part of a polygenic system that governs the same complex function. If so, it is not unexpected that environmental factors could influence the pathogenesis of these tumors as well. All of these features will make it difficult to identify homologous genes in man. However, the localization of a gene in the mouse may permit identification of homologous locus in man through syntenic groups. Further identification one polygene may reveal to identifying a network of genes (Laurie-Ahlberg et al. 1980) that are related to a common regulatory function such as a signal transduction pathway involved controlling growth.

REFERENCES

Anderson AO, Wax JW, Potter M (1985) Differences in the peritoneal response to pristane in BALB/cAnPt and BALB/cJ mice. In: Potter M (ed) Current topics in microbiology and immunology, vol. 122. Springer, Berlin Heidelberg New York, pp 242-253

Anderson PN, Potter M (1969) Induction of plasma cell tumors in BALB/c mice with 2,6,10,14-tetramethylpentadecane (pristane). Nature 222:994-995

Brandt SJ, Bodine DM, Dunbar CE, Nienhuis AW (1990) Retroviral-mediated transfer of interleukin-6 into hematopoietic cells of mice results in a syndrome resembling Castleman's disease. In: Potter M, Melchers F (eds) Current topics in microbiology and immunology. Springer, Berlin Heidelberg New York, in press

Cillari E, Liew FY, Lelchuk R (1986) Suppression of interleukin-2 production by macrophages in genetically susceptible mice infected with Leishmania major. Infect Immun 54:386-394

Goldings EA (1986) Regulation of B-cell tolerance by macrophage-derived mediators: antagonistic effects of prostaglandin E2 and interleukin 1. J Imm 136:817-822

Goodwin JS, Bankhurst AD, Messner RP (1977) Suppression of human T-cell mitogenesis by prostaglandin. J Exp Med 146:1719-1734

Jelinek DF, Thompson PA, Lipsky PE (1985) Regulation of human B cell actiation by prostaglandin E2. Suppression of the generation of immunoglobulin secreting cells. J Clin Invest 75:1339-1349

Laurie-Ahlberg CC, Maroni G, Bewley GC, Lucchesi JC, Weir BS (1980) Quantitative genetic variation of enzyme activities in natural populations of Drosophila melanogaster. Proc Natl Acad Sci USA 77:1073-1077

Leak LV, Potter M, Mayfield WJ (1985) Response of the peritoneal mesothelium to the mineral oil pristane. In: Potter M (ed) Current topics in microbiology and immunology, vol. 122. Springer, Berlin Heidelberg New York, pp 221-233

Liew FY (19) Suppressor cells for cell-mediated immunity in infectious diseases. 26th Forum in Immunology, pp 328-333

Liew FY (1990) Regulation of cell-mediated immunity in Leishmaniasis. In: Kaufmann SHE (ed) Current topics in microbiology and immunology, vol 155. T-cell paradigms in parasitic and bacterial infections. Springer, Berlin Heidelberg New York, pp 53-64

Merwin RM, Redmon LW (1963) Induction of plasma cell tumors and sarcomas in mice by diffusion chambers placed in the peritoneal cavity. J Natl Cancer Inst 31:998-1007

Morse HC III, Hartley JW, Potter M (1980) Genetic considerations in plasmacytomas of BALB/c NZB and (BALB/c x NZB)F1 mice. In: Potter M (ed) Progress in myeloma. Biology of myeloma. Elsevier, North Holland New York, p 263

Ohno S, Babonits M, Wiener F, et al (1979) Non-random chromosome changes involving the Ig gene-carrying chromosomes 12 and 6 in pristane-induced mouse plasmacytomas. Cell 18:1001-1007

Ohno S, Migita S, Wiener F, Babonits M, Klein G, Mushinski JF, Potter M (1984) Chromosomal translocations activating myc sequences and transduction of v-abl are critical events in the rapid induction of plasmacytomas by pristane and Abelson virus. J Exp Med 159:1762-1777

Phipps RP, Lee D, Schad V, Warner GL (1989) E-series prostaglandins are potent growth inhibitors for some B lymphomas. Eur J Immunol 19:995-1001

McIntire KR, Princler GL (1969) Prolonged adjuvant stimulation in germ-free BALB/c ,development of plasma cell neoplasia. Immunology 17:481-487

Potter M, MacCardle RC (1964) Histology of developing plasma cell neoplasia induced by mineral oil in BALB/c mice. J Natl Cancer Inst 33:497

Potter M, Walters JL (1973) Effects of intraperitoneal pristane on established immunity to the Adj-PC-5 plasmacytoma. J Natl Cancer Inst 51:875-881

Potter M, Wax JS, Anderson AO, Nordan RP (1985) Inhibition of plasmacytoma development in BALB/c mice by indomethacin. J Exp Med 161:996-1012

Potter M, Wax JS (1983) Peritoneal plasmacytomagenesis in mice. A comparison of three pristane dose regimens. J Natl Cancer Inst 71:391

Potter M, Pumphrey JG, Bailey DW (1975) Genetics of susceptibility of plasmacytomas induction. I. BALB/cAnN (C), C57BL/6N (B6), C57BL/Ka (BK), (C x B6)F1 (C x BK)F1 and C x B recombinant inbred strains. J Natl Cancer Inst 54:1413

Potter M (1984) Genetics of susceptibility to plasmacytoma development in BALB/c mice. Cancer Surveys 3:247-264

Potter M, Hartley JW, Wax JS and Gallahan D (1984) Effect of MuLV-related genes on plasmacytomagenesis in BALB/c mice. J Exp Med 160:435-440

Potter M, Wax JS (1986) Inbred strain differences influence the focal proliferation of plasma cells in prostane induced oil granuloma. In: Melchers F, Potter M (eds) Current Topics in Microbiology and Immunology, vol. 132. Springer, Berlin Heidelberg New York, pp 227-230

Radl J (1981) Animal model of human disease. Benign monoclonal gammopathy (idiopathic paraproteinemia). Am J Pathol 105:91

Rincon M, Tugores A, Lopez-Rivas A, Silva A, Alonso M, DeLandazuri MO, Lopez-Botet M (1988) Prostaglandin E2 and the increase of intracellular cAMP inhibit the expression of interleukin 2 receptors in human T cells. Eur J Immunol 18:1791-1796

Rojo JM, Portoles MP, Barasoain I, Portoles A (1982) Exogenous additions of prostaglandins variably alter the blastogenic response of B and T lymphocytes from different mice lymphoid organs. Immunopharmacology 4:95-104

Scheuer WV, Hobbs MV, Weigle WO (1987) Interference with tolerance induction in vivo by inhibitors of prostaglandin synthesis. Cell Immunol 104:409-418

Schad V, Phipps RP (1989) Prostaglandin E2-dependent induction of B cell unresponsiveness: role of surface Ig and Fc receptors. J Immunol 143:2127-2132

Suematsu S, Matsuda T, Aozasa K, Akira S, Nakano N, Ohno S, Miyazaki J-I, Yamamura K-I, Hirano T, Kishimoto T (1989) IgG1 plasmacytosis in interleukin 6 transgenic mice. Proc Natl Acad Sci USA 86:7547-7551

Weiss S, Lehmann K, Raschke WC, Cohn M (1984) Mice completely suppressed for the expression of immunoglobulin k light chain. Proc Natl Acad Sci USA 81:211-215

MIX
Papier aus verantwortungsvollen Quellen
Paper from responsible sources
FSC® C105338

If you have any concerns about our products,
you can contact us on
ProductSafety@springernature.com

In case Publisher is established outside the EU,
the EU authorized representative is:
Springer Nature Customer Service Center GmbH
Europaplatz 3, 69115 Heidelberg, Germany

Printed by Libri Plureos GmbH
in Hamburg, Germany